DEDICATION

I acknowledge my indebtedness to the thousands of DOs who came before me.
Through their influence, organized activity and persistence, they advanced the osteopathic profession to the point where I could stand on their shoulders.

AND

I acknowledge my indebtedness to my peers and colleagues who, either alone or in concert with others, gave their all to continue to advance the osteopathic profession.

AND

I acknowledge my indebtedness to all the thousands of DOs who came after me and carried the baton forward to advance even further the osteopathic profession.

They brought us to today's status of acceptance and recognition.
To all of them I say a heartfelt "Thank You!"

OTHER BOOKS BY THE AUTHOR

Pediatrics: Some Uncommon Views on Some Common Problems

Professionally Speaking: Public Speaking for Health Professionals

Oratoris para Profesionales de la Salud (Professionally Speaking)

Medical Writing 101: A Primer for Health Professionals

Parenthood: Laugh and Understand Your Child

Ethical Problems in Pediatrics: A Dozen Dilemmas

Effective Medical Communication: An Anthology of Columns

Looking Back . . . at SECOM

Practicing for Practice

Melnick on Writing

MONOGRAPHS

So, you've been asked to speak . . .

Sandy, We Love You (with Anita Melnick)

Who Will I Tell?

Osteopathic Tales

Stories tracing one DO's travel along the path of the Osteopathic Profession from Rejection and Discrimination to Recognition and Acceptance

Arnold Melnick
DO, MSc, DHL (HON.), FACOP

authorHOUSE®

AuthorHouse™
1663 Liberty Drive
Bloomington, IN 47403
www.authorhouse.com
Phone: 1-800-839-8640

Published by AuthorHouse 03/18/2013

ISBN: 978-1-4817-3224-6 (sc)
ISBN: 978-1-4817-3223-9 (e)

Library of Congress Control Number: 2013905134

This book is printed on acid-free paper.

CONTENTS

PART TWO
Early Practice . . . and Beyond

PART THREE
The Merger

PART FOUR
The CHOP Years

PART FIVE
Writing and Speaking

PART SIX
The SECOM Years

Preface

I GRADUATED FROM THE Philadelphia College of Osteopathy (now the Philadelphia College of Osteopathic Medicine) in 1945. Even though I had some inkling that it existed, I was met by a world of hostility and rejection as an osteopathic physician.

Osteopathic Tales is a collection of true anecdotes that occurred during the long period of the profession's rise in acceptance and recognition. Most are personal experiences and observations, some involve other people, and a few are gratuitous stories that were worth including. But most are examples of steps that occurred throughout the country in the great progression of osteopathic medicine over my professional lifetime, a period of 65+years.

So the stories in this book are half-autobiographical, half-historical and half illustrative of that climb. (You'll see how much overlap there is.) These tales illustrate, for the most part, the human side of the struggle.

Thankfully, over these many years, the atmosphere has totally changed and there is now widespread acceptance and recognition of DOs—by the allopathic profession and all federal, state and local governmental agencies, as well as the entire population.

As all this happened, our osteopathic colleges were expanding from 5 in 1945 to 30 colleges and branches today—with yearly graduating classes of under 400 in 1945 increasing to almost 5,000 now, and with almost 10,000 approved residency training positions. The number of DOs has grown from 10,000+ in the entire country to over 77,000 now. In 1945, a number of states still limited the practice rights of DOs, but by 1973, every state and the District of Columbia licensed DOs for full-practice rights.

I am grateful for the tremendous progress that occurred, grateful for the wider role played by the osteopathic profession in the medical world and grateful for the opportunity accorded me to have lived through this fantastic phenomenon.

The number of personal references was unavoidable but were meant to exemplify what was going on throughout the osteopathic profession and being experienced by many other members of our profession.

—*Arnold Melnick, DO*

INTRODUCTION

I HAD ADEQUATE MEDICAL training in my four academic years at PCO and it well prepared me for practice. Some vintage observers may challenge that adequacy, but medical schools (including osteopathic) have always had varying degrees of adequacy and many different curricula and they cannot always be compared. All schools produce competent doctors (with a few wayward ones). While there may have been a few inadequate areas, such as extensive clinical experience, PCO (and other osteopathic colleges) did produce fine physicians.

One of the obvious shortcomings was the lack of enough graduate training opportunities, so the majority of DOs went into what was called General Practice (now named Family Medicine). Opportunities to become specialists were very limited, even though a number of DOs did manage to get enough graduate training to go into specialty practice. There were opportunities for residency training in surgery at several osteopathic hospitals, and a scattered few other specialty residencies. Many (not all) of our graduates did serve one-year internships. But the bulk of the profession was general practice.

Those osteopathic physicians who went into specialty practice other than surgery had trained surreptitiously, taking their training through some of the few courses that were open to them or working with willing individual specialists (both allopathic and osteopathic) who acted as preceptors.

Gradually, over these years, the number of DOs rose dramatically, osteopathic residencies proliferated, more osteopathic hospitals developed, graduate training grew and the profession produced more and more specialists.

During that growth (from mid-century on), occasional openings arose for a DO here and there to get allopathic specialty training and toward the end of the century many allopathic hospitals and training programs opened their doors to osteopathic physicians and they were accepted. Ultimately, even a number of allopathic specialty boards allowed DOs to take specialty certification examinations along with their MD colleagues (in addition to osteopathic certifying boards), and state boards allowed MDs and DOs to take the same examinations—together. Today, a great number of allopathic hospitals (among them some of the most highly regarded institutions in this country) have DOs as active staff members. And DOs serve as department heads in medical schools and chiefs in allopathic hospitals.

Osteopathic Tales is a collection of interesting and illustrative stories that occurred during that stretch of time—while showing how the profession grew and became accepted. Some names have been left out in order not to embarrass anyone, some quotations are actually reconstructions or paraphrasing; in some instances the time sequences are the way I remember them and may not be sequential—but all of them are true and factual.

Since these tales are those I encountered in a 70-year period, there is an unavoidable tendency to be autobiographical. If I crossed the line at any point, I apologize. Many DOs had comparable experiences.

Status of Osteopathy

1942-1945

To the best of my recollection, this section represents the status of the profession (then called "osteopathy" and now called "osteopathic medicine") at the time I attended Philadelphia College of Osteopathic Medicine in 1942-1945. While memories of 70 years ago sometimes have soft spots, I feel certain that the representation here is an accurate picture of the profession.

Medical Education. PCO was a four-year course, in our case three calendar years into which was compressed a four-year curriculum because of the on-going war. Like all other DO schools, PCO required at least 90 undergraduate credit hours for admission, adhering to the recommendation of the Flexner Report (which guided all allopathic schools). The first two years were devoted to laboratory and classroom learning in basic medical sciences, and then two years of introductory clinical courses and experience. These were the same curricular guidelines followed by all allopathic medical schools.

The educational arm of osteopathy had a total of only six osteopathic medical schools which were very much similar to PCO—a few with attached hospitals and others without. That amounted to a total of a couple of hundred osteopathic students in osteopathic colleges.

The number of female osteopathic students (like the number of female DOs then in practice) was infinitesimal. In my PCO class, there was one female (out of 45), and I would estimate that in the entire four-year complement of students at PCO, there were fewer than five females.

Faculty. This was composed almost entirely of osteopathic physicians, with a very occasional MD instructor. In the basic sciences, we had both DO and PhD teachers. In the clinical fields, our classes were taught by DOs who were totally competent in their fields and usually were practicing specialists. Like in all allopathic and osteopathic schools, a few were not up to par; some were good and others outstanding.

Post-Graduate. There were only a few osteopathic training hospitals in the U.S.—and, of course, no allopathic hospitals were available to DOs. Since many states did not require post-graduate training for state licensure, many (most?) of our graduates went directly from graduation into what was then called General Practice (and most were successful at it). In my graduating class (1945) of 43 DOs, roughly 13 were able to obtain osteopathically-approved internships; a few were successful in getting internships/residencies at unapproved hospitals, especially in New York. (Fortunately, they did get training). Specialty training was even further limited, and was mainly surgical. And most DOs who went into surgical training often had to act as general residents because there were no other residents around. PCO's Osteopathic Hospital of Philadelphia, arguably a leader in our profession, had one surgical residency available each year; its first Internal Medicine residency (one person) began in 1947, as did the first Pediatrics residency (also one person). In some aspects of this training, some osteopathic hospitals were ahead of us, notably in Michigan.

Licensure. Many of the states granted licensure (by examination) upon graduation, but there were, until a few years ago, a couple of states that had limited licensure for DOs. And I have a vague memory that a few states did not license osteopaths at all. For example, Pennsylvania for many year required additional training and examination for a DO to be licensed as a surgeon—so it was in reality a limited license. That law was changed in the 1950s. By 1973, all states and the District of Columbia fully licensed DOs.

Recognition and acceptance. In none of this period was osteopathy recognized or accepted by any AMA—connected organization or institution—nor by the Armed Forces. Government jobs (local, state and federal were likewise not available to DOs). Most civilian opportunities seemed to follow AMA policies, cutting off any potential employment for osteopaths. Our opportunities were quite restricted.

So, facing us on graduation was the choice: beg, borrow or steal as much graduate training as we could get or go into General Practice.

I chose both. I worked part time in a senior physician's office, doing whatever came along, but I concentrated on the PCO Preceptor Program in Pediatrics for my training, in addition to whatever I could "pick up." After one year, I limited my private practice to Pediatrics (even without formal training). Under this regime, I became trained and certified in Pediatrics.

This is where I entered the osteopathic profession and began to collect memories.

(Please also see **Status of Osteopathic Medicine, 2013,** *on Page 153.)*

PART ONE

The Early Days

UPON COMPLETING MY internship, I went into private general practice, as the osteopathic profession only had two pediatric residencies (and they were in California). But my drive always was to become qualified in Pediatrics, so a lot of my time was spent seeking out pediatric conferences and courses that I was allowed (or not allowed) to attend, but I devoted most of my time (besides my practice) to the Pediatric Preceptorship offered at my alma mater under the direction, first of Ruth Tinley, DO, FACOP, and mostly under William S. Spaeth, DO, FACOP, who succeeded Dr. Tinley as Department Chair. Several of us enrolled in this program, and we spent four hours a week in the Pediatrics Clinic under the tutelage of Dr. Spaeth, F. Munro Purse, DO, FACOP, and Harry Breitman, DO, FACOP, plus doing ward rounds in the PCO Hospital with the Attending Staff.

These tales arose mostly during that time (approximately 1946-1950).

TALE 1

Chasing Courses

ONE OF THE major routes we sought for training was specific, short courses offered by medical schools or hospitals. I—and many of my colleagues—kept our eyes open for such opportunities, even though we knew that rarely was a DO welcome to attend. We took our chances.

Such an opportunity arose for me. I saw an advertisement in one of the medial journals for a course in pediatric development given by Arnold Gesell, MD, of Yale University, a world-renowned researcher and clinician. What an opening—but how would I get in? And would they take me?

Using the major subterfuge used by many DOs at that time, I did register for the course. But I registered as Arnold Melnick, MD. I had to take the chance. Luckily, I was accepted. It meant traveling to New

Haven ten Mondays, as I recall, at a tuition cost of $150. Expensive (for then) but I had to go.

So off I went that first Monday. I flew into New Haven, taxied to Yale and went to the appointed auditorium. As I approached the door, I noticed a small group of people standing around a table right at the entrance. I wasn't going to take a chance, so I waited until they dispersed, and then cautiously approached. There on the table was a signature book, with the request for registrants to sign in. Not me, I was an imposter; I even felt like a criminal. I by-passed the desk and the sign-in book and went into the first day's session.

On subsequent Mondays, I was careful to avoid signing in—I didn't want to get caught. Imagine having that panicky feeling when all I wanted to do was learn. But it was worth the suffering. And I was most successful in evading registering. And I learned a great deal. And I was thrilled to learn literally at the feet of a brilliant physician, one of our earliest and most well-known developmentalists. My subterfuge had worked.

Smug and self-satisfied—and armed with the latest information on childhood development, I went back to my everyday routines. Content—that is, until a few weeks later, when I received in the mail an envelope from the Gesell Institute at Yale, addressed to Arnold Melnick, <u>MD.</u>

Was it an advertisement? A thank-you for attending? I ripped it open and found a brief letter, signed by Dr. Gesell himself. It read something like this:

> Dear Dr. Melnick:
>
> We are sorry that you were unable to attend our recent course at Yale. Enclosed is a check for $150, your returned tuition.
>
> /s/ Arnold Gesell, MD

I kept that check—uncashed—as a souvenir but the financial pressures of a beginning practice forced me to deposit it after a few days—reluctantly but gleefully.

This was one of the subterfuges we had to use to obtain graduate education.

TALE 2

. . . and another Course

THIS TIME, IT was another course—one at George Washington University School of Medicine and it was scheduled for several days. It seemed most interesting, so I decided to apply—again using Arnold Melnick, with an MD after my name. But this time, they wanted to know what medical school I graduated from and in what year. I was non-plussed. Then suddenly, it struck me. I had a cousin, a Melnick who was a year behind me and who graduated from Jefferson Medical College.

So I took the risk, using my full name, using the MD degree, and using his school and year of graduation—constantly hoping that they would not discover the difference in first names. They didn't.

Once again, on arrival I saw a group of physicians gathered around a bulletin board, obviously something to do with the course. Again, I waited and found posted a list of registrants. And there I was on that list. Just the way I applied: with Jefferson and 1946 next to my name. A sudden panic hit me—suppose there was another Jefferson graduate from around the same time? I didn't scan the list, I devoured it. Thank goodness, no one from that school—someone who could possibly identify this imposter.

I entered the auditorium and enjoyed the course. And, once more, all this subterfuge in order to gain a little learning. This is the way it was with almost all of the outside training that I—and hundreds of other DOs—sought, and often were fortunately successful.

Sometimes we were lucky. One of my goals was to learn some pediatric psychiatry. I noted a course being given locally by the Philadelphia Psychoanalytic Society. I knew not what they stood for or what their opinion of osteopathic medicine was, but I thought I would take a chance: I applied, using my DO degree—and was accepted. I learned a lot in that course and at that point I didn't care whether they were way ahead of the rest of the medical world by allowing DOs into the course, or whether they had some other motivation, but I was overjoyed to find an MD course open to me—and a chance to add to my knowledge. In retrospect it was another small step for the osteopathic profession.

TALE 3

Two More "Course" Tales

TWO MORE STORIES about courses and the problems associated with them.

It was in the sixties, and Harold Finkel, DO, FACOP, in Lancaster, PA, Martyn E. Richardson, DO, FACOP, in St. Louis, and I in Philadelphia noticed almost simultaneously that the Mayo Clinic was presenting an interesting three-day course in Pediatric Neurology. We got out heads together and decided to apply. And, if I remember correctly, we applied as DOs—and were accepted. Apparently (I hoped), they had already recognized the progress of Osteopathic Medicine.

The course was being given by Manny Perez, MD, a young, energetic and talented member of Mayo's staff who treated us with total equality—I don't remember any time that the subject of Osteopathic Medicine even came up in speaking with him. There were perhaps 60 or so registrants and the course was fascinating and packed with learning.

Also in attendance was a small group of MD pediatricians from Texas who repeatedly complained about "the damned osteopaths back home." There was a dinner at the closing of the course, and all participants were introduced—with their degrees. It was reported that the complaining MDs were red-faced when they found out that they had been working with three DOs all week.

Poetic justice!

Miami Children's Hospital annually ran a huge Pediatric Refresher Course, each year attracting over 1000 participants. They presented a host of national and international pediatric experts ("names") and ran the program with carefully timed and controlled lectures. Each year it was a magnificent graduate course.

One of my local friends, an MD pediatrician who practiced a few blocks from me, and I decided to attend. When we got to the meeting in Miami, I found six or seven other DO pediatricians (all of them my friends) who were also there. Of course, I introduced him to my friends. It was "Dr. Rosenberg, this is my colleague, Dr . . . . (name of the DO)."

Near the end of the meeting Dr. Rosenberg turned to me and said, "Arnold, how come there are a thousand MDs here and I don't know a single one. But there is only a handful of DOs and you know every one?" He was embarrassed.

But he had discovered one of our secrets. Not only was it because of the much smaller number of DOs totally and thus fewer DO pediatricians but, as I always said. "Although we were a profession, we also were a close-knit fraternity . . . a brotherhood, if you will."

TALE 4

Dealing with Pharmaceutical Companies

IN THE MID-CENTURY years, osteopathic physicians and osteopathic organizations found other sources of discrimination—some were pharmaceutical companies. There were many reasons. Numerically, the DO profession was very small, so their contribution to a company's business was not significant. Then, too, most such companies had an MD Medical Director or MD researchers—their outlook followed the mode of the day: anti-osteopathic or at least semi-anti-osteopathic And always, there were overt and subtle pressures on them from certain allopathic groups.

As always, a great source of income for osteopathic organizations (and allopathic ones, too) was the sale of exhibit space at medical meetings. I was at the time of this incident (1958) President of the Pennsylvania Osteopathic Association (now the Pennsylvania

Osteopathic Medical Association—POMA). The "detail man" from a major pharmaceutical company that had turned us down for an exhibit came to my office to "detail" me; I refused to see him and told him why. (And yes, they did call on DOs, even though not recognizing them officially.)

It was interesting that we received reports that visits to DOs were more productive than visits to MDs—better good-will and more prescriptions for each "detail" visit. But we were still small in total.

Not long after that, he made a special appointment to see me with a higher-up in his company (General Manager? Vice President?). The senior representative made a nice presentation, explaining about limited funds, the need to place their money in the most strategic spots, small attendance at osteopathic meetings, and so forth. My counter: I told him that I understood but felt that some support should be shown to the many DOs who did write for their company's products and we felt that they were not supportive.

After 10 or 15 minutes of quiet, non-confrontational discussion, the "boss" pulled his big gun, something like this, "Our company has an increase in business income of nearly 10% every year. Osteopathic physicians account for barely 5% of our business. So, if every DO stopped writing for our products, the company would never notice it." I was furious at his brash, insulting statement.

Rather than getting embroiled in a vociferous argument, I chose the smarter path. I said, "OK, if that's the way you feel and the way you want to operate, thank you for coming to see me." With that, I stood up and he knew the meeting was over.

I knew that boycotts were illegal, so I couldn't threaten one or do one. But I took a different approach—sort of a reverse one. I immediately circulated to all DOs in the state a list of those companies (with much praise) who were supporting the osteopathic profession by exhibiting and had signed up for the coming convention. I also suggested subtly that all DOs do what they could to convince the recalcitrant companies to come aboard. I wasn't really sure whether it would do any good.

About two to three weeks later, the executive called for another appointment. I made one for him. His opening gambit, hostilely, was, "What's all this nonsense that's going on?" I pleaded ignorance of what he was talking about. He railed that no Pennsylvania DO would allow his representative to enter the office. I simply shrugged my shoulders to which he said, angrily, "OK, we'll take a booth!"

And that company has been with POMA ever since.

This was one of many machinations we had to go through to get support from a number of suppliers—and almost all of that discrimination from drug companies is gone today.

Tale 5

Another Drug Company Tale

Another problem. Another drug company. Another solution.

One day, I noticed a Wyeth Laboratories advertisement in one of the pediatric journals announcing the availability of financial support, via a stipend, for pediatric residents. Interesting, except that one of the requirements was possession of an MD degree. At that time, we had just started our Pediatrics residency at PCO.

Once more, the hair on my neck stood up and I dispatched a letter to the president of Wyeth. I later learned from outside (or inside) sources that he immediately gave it to one of his vice-presidents. That vice-president then turned to a young detail representative named Justin McCarthy, with the comment supposedly, "Go see this guy. Give him a few samples and get him off of our back."

That was my introduction to Justin McCarthy. He called on me. A perfect gentleman. We discussed the matter and he understood, and promised to take our message back to company officials. Meanwhile, Justin and I became friends on a personal basis: his son and my son both were attending the University of Rochester. We met there and we became rather close.

There was no dramatic ending to this story. I believe that Wyeth explained to us that they had set up a two-year program. Somehow the program disappeared, promptly at the end of the initial two years. Either it didn't work out or it was easier to discontinue than to add DOs to the program.

What did work out was Justin McCarthy's interest in and eventually dedication to the osteopathic profession. Over the years, as he was rising within the company, he became active in various aspects of our profession and ultimately served as President of the National Osteopathic Foundation.

Apparently, from that time on, and mostly because of the strong support from my brother DOs, Wyeth could be counted on to assist our DO organizations.

Another victory, but not the way I would have liked it. But I'll take winning whatever way I can get it. It helped strengthen the osteopathic profession. Our group gained another supporter. And especially because Justin came along with the deal.

Tale 6

An Earlier Kind of Discrimination

I have to reach back to include another, an earlier kind of discrimination that affected doctors and prospective doctors in those early days—before I graduated. And it had a bearing on the osteopathic profession.

In 1940-41, I was a pre-medical student at Temple University, doing the usual thing—filing applications, searching for a medical school acceptance, and in some instances undergoing interviews.

I was unlucky, I didn't get a single medical (allopathic) acceptance. Disturbed and perplexed about this, my father, who was an outstanding salesman, decided to take the bull by the horns. He made an appointment to see William Parkinson, MD, who was the Dean at Temple Medical School at the time.

My father made an eloquent plea, outlining all the reasons he thought I should have been accepted, and, of course, praised me beyond all measure. Dr. Parkinson listed attentively and quietly and let my father speak.

When the "pitch" was finished, Dr. Parkinson softly and non-hostilely said to my father, "Mr. Melnick, even if your son were everything you say he is, I could not admit him. You see, we already have our quota of Jews for this year." It was said as a simple matter of fact.

Startling? No. It was school policy, one that existed in many medical—and other professional—schools. And it applied not only to Jews but other minorities—blacks and Italians and women in particular. It was overt and unhidden. Numerical quota were in style and accepted. Discrimination existed openly everywhere—well, almost everywhere.

With civil rights rising in the public's conscience and with discrimination being held up to the light everywhere, this then-accepted custom gradually faded and then disappeared. Some believe that it may still exist in some schools but sub-rosa. It probably reflects the rise of fairness in American life and policies—a movement long in coming but most welcome.

Luckily for me, I discovered osteopathic medicine—PCO in particular. I became a doctor—proudly an osteopathic one—and started my medical career. It went far beyond my dreams: it gave me full medical practice rights, pediatrics training, access to untold riches of personal and professional contacts, and a life most rewarding and appreciated.

So what does this have to do with the growth of osteopathic medicine? Erwin A. Blackstone, professor of economics at Temple University wrote "A Tale of Two Doctors" in *Regulation* (Summer, 2010, p. 7) describing the two professions, MD and DO, and established "the substantial benefits society derives from having a small competitor that helps constrain the power of organized allopathic medicine"—giving economics credence to what has happened with osteopathic medicine and allopathic medicine. In that piece, he also says, ". . . when discrimination in the 1930s and 1940s prevented many Jewish applicants from becoming MDs, many chose to become DOs. Jewish enrollment in osteopathic medical schools increased from 9.1 percent to 20.3 percent between 1935 and 1946, largely attributable to their being discriminated against in admission to MD schools." Simultaneously, the same phenomenon was happening to other to other discrimination victims—blacks, Italians, women. The entering classes at osteopathic colleges started to grow, more and more families and friends of those students became acquainted with osteopathic medicine. And many of them found good medical care, liked it and stayed on as osteopathic patients.

The good word about Osteopathic Medicine was spreading to newer and larger groups and the osteopathic profession was on its way.

So count me as one of them—another cog in the wheel of advancement.

TALE 7

Drafting Doctors (MDs) Helped

TALES FROM THE rise of the osteopathic profession are interesting and sometimes fascinating, and they are examples of the profession's fight for obtaining equity. They gained us recognition from official governmental agencies and from commercial sources. But they did not put patients into DO's waiting rooms!

Probably different people place emphasis on different forces as giving the profession increasing numbers of patients—and with it, acceptance as full-fledged physicians.

One phenomenon cannot be overlooked. It was evident in the 1940s.

At the time I graduated (1945), World War II was ending. Most of us in osteopathic schools received deferments from the draft to complete our medical studies. But an interesting situation was playing out. The allopathic profession, backed by allopathic organizations, and powered by MD leaders in the armed-services Medical Corps, declared osteopathic physicians to be "quacks", unqualified to serve in the armed services as physicians, so we were not eligible for commissions. So for the entire war, no DO held a commission as a physician. A few who were drafted rather than deferred were assigned as medical corpsmen.

(Today, that discrimination is gone; our DOs are totally eligible. In fact, just a few years ago, Ronald R. Blank, DO, served as Surgeon-General of the U.S. Army, after a term as Commanding General of Walter Reed Hospital.)

So our graduating DOs went into private practice, mostly as general practitioners. Some (the lucky ones) served one-year internships, and then opened private offices. Overwhelmingly, that is what DO graduates did.

What a situation! MDs were being drafted out of their practice or out of residencies, up to the age of 50 or 55, tremendously diminishing the supply of MD physicians in civilian life serving the general public. Entire neighborhoods were bereft of physicians. Closed offices were everywhere. Meanwhile, increasing numbers of osteopathic physicians were opening offices and being available for seeing patients.

What happened?

Patients seeking medical care had lost their doctors (MDs) and their doctor's colleagues were gone, too.

Many patients were desperate. People talk. A neighbor, or friend, or relative, hearing of the distress, responded in one of several ways, such as:

> "My doctor is a DO and I get great care. Why don't you call him?"
>
> "I had the same problem; my physician was drafted. I was referred to this DO and I find that he's a regular doctor. I recommend him"

Many patients found competent care, holistic medicine and genuine personal interest—and when the crush was over, they remained loyal osteopathic patients. (It is probably redundant to say that half the credit here goes to the DOs whose splendid medical care convinced the new patients that they were real doctors.) Of course, some patients retained feelings for their first doctor, or many preferred the old "doc" (and returned to them), but a landslide of patients became patients of the osteopathic physicians—almost by necessity—and many of them stayed.

Literally, the patient load of DOs increased tremendously because of the absence of the drafted MDs. Even the newly-minted DOs were able to build practices very fast.

Thus, this discrimination against DOs by the armed forced backfired. It led to a shortage of civilian MD doctors, and hordes of patients were essentially forced to use osteopathic physicians. Many of these patients appeared to be happy—or at least satisfied—and DO practices flourished. So this MD discrimination actually helped the osteopathic profession to grow. And as these practices grew, many of the satisfied patients referred families and friends to DOs.

This anomalous situation was in great part responsible for the rapid acceleration of the growth of the osteopathic profession by creating innumerable patients available for osteopathic physicians.

Tale 8

Growth of Osteopathic Hospitals

Another great boost to osteopathic acceptance and recognition—slowly, of course—was the growth and development of osteopathic hospitals. There was no master plan, no program for creating new hospitals. Like Topsy, they "jest growed". When the growth of osteopathic practice in an area cried out for a hospital where they could treat their patients, the DOs would get together and establish a small hospital—no government assistance, no community financial help and no outside stimuli or help. They just used their own money. Everything came from the profession itself.

When I went into practice, Philadelphia had one major osteopathic hospital, part of PCO, and a small developing hospital, Metropolitan Hospital. Chicago, likewise, as a part of the Chicago College of Osteopathy. Detroit you might say was a hub; it had two—Detroit Osteopathic Hospital and Art Centre Hospital. In

Michigan, there were a couple of other osteopathic hospitals and Michigan was sort of looked upon as an icon of osteopathic graduate education. A few other scattered hospitals did exist and contributed to the growth of the profession as well as the far-thinking DOs who established and maintained them. This brief summary barely brushes the development situation and many early osteopathic hospitals could be cited.

Within a few years, a new osteopathic hospital sprung up here and there. You must remember that allopathic hospitals did not train DOs, and did not give DOs admitting privileges Many DOs admitted their patients to DO hospitals, if there were any close by, and cared for them themselves; DO general practitioners treated their own hospitalized patients, utilizing whatever specialists were available. Otherwise, they would lose their patients to allopathic hospitals.

The profession was in a situation where, slowly but surely, more and more hospitals were springing up. And one or two at a time, surgeons were being trained, and internists as well, and that's about all. But these newly-trained specialists either came from another hospital and planned to return there as fully-accredited specialists or looked for an osteopathic hospital that could use their services. Once again, they were not permitted to work in allopathic hospitals.

As a result of this situation, osteopathic hospitals expanded into other needed specialty fields that arose and hospitals grew further. Surgeons and internists were the initial backbone of new osteopathic hospitals (many of them quite small), and with the rise of other specialties—radiology and pathology, for starters—the hospitals grew further.

With all this unplanned growth, more and more patients were being hospitalized in osteopathic institutions. And patients were finding that osteopathic care was excellent and current. The cycle kept spinning until the latter part of the century when osteopathic hospitals were more plentiful and the public was getting more exposed to DOs. As a result there was great acceptance by the public. And the allopathic profession had to take notice. Inter-professional and inter-hospital consultations were occurring more frequently.

A secondary effect of the growth of osteopathic hospitals, in size and complexity, is that more potential patients were exposed to our profession and, maybe more important, more and more potential students were exposed to osteopathic medicine and what it offered.

This brief survey hardly does justice to the tremendous hospital growth in our profession and its fantastic effect on the acceptance and recognition of the osteopathic profession. I am so grateful that I lived through this period and glad to offer accolades to the many colleagues involved in it. I am certainly glad that I was able to see this phenomenon.

(However, with the late-century acceptance of osteopathic physicians, the ability of DOs to hospitalize their patients in major allopathic hospitals and a number of osteopathic physicians working exclusively in allopathic hospitals, there followed a dying-off of many osteopathic hospitals and the total number of them diminished greatly. A boon or bane? Only the future will be able to tell accurately.)

Tale 9

Minority of a Minority

One of the very noticeable characteristics of the physician population—in both the allopathic and osteopathic professions—around the 1940s was the tiny number of female physicians. For example, in my medical school class of 40 students, there was one female. As I recall, in all my medical school days—three years before me and three years after me—perhaps there were a half-dozen ladies-in-training. Medicine was not a profession loaded with the female gender; there were few female applicants, few acceptances and few gr aduates. In the osteopathic profession, they were truly a minority of a minority

Since those days, things have changed—more female applicants, more acceptances and more graduates. Just look at what has happened in recent years. The population of women in our profesasion has gradually increased. Take 1969 as an in-between year (actually the climb began earlier than that): there were just under 2000 registered osteopathic students (all four classes), and that year a total of 427 graduated from osteopathic colleges; only a handful of them were women. By 2010, the group had exploded: 19,427 students, with a graduating class that year of 3,631, about half of them women. Actually, female students have now constituted around 50% for a number of years.

Osteopathic medicine has grown tremendously since my day, and the female number has expanded geometrically. The same is true of allopathic medicine and I know this metamorphosis has made a great impact on the practice of medicine.

An unusual personification of the female physician in the early 20th century was Ruth E. Tinley, DO, mentioned earlier. She was my first professor of pediatrics. An Ethel Barrymore—type lady, she was a fine pediatrician, friendly and warm—a grandmother figure. But when crossed, she could stand her ground. I liked her. She was one of the founders of the American College of Osteopathic Pediatricians and served as its second president, in 1943.

Dr. Tinley always had some interesting stories to tell. One, above all, stood out and whenever she told it, she had to laugh again—it drew the picture of the public perception of female physicians.

These were the days of "house calls." Dr. Tinley was called to see a young boy too sick to come to the office. She took the history from the mother and did a thorough examination of the little lad. As she finished and gave the mother instructions, the boy turned to his mother and asked, "Wasn't that nice of the doctor?" Anxious to let Dr. Tinley hear some praise from her patient, the mother asked, "Wasn't what nice?" Without hesitation, the youngster replied, "The doctor couldn't come, so he sent his mother."

How things have changed since then!

Commentary

It is worth noting again the great influence of factors that contributed much to the growth and eventual acceptance of the osteopathic profession:

1. The discrimination of allopathic school in the early years in the admission of certain minorities: Jews, blacks, Italians and women. These groups then discovered osteopathic medicine and flocked to our profession.
2. The discrimination of the armed forces during World War II that kept DOs from service as medical officers, leaving the DOs at home, and literally sending thousands of patients to DOs.
3. The growth of osteopathic hospitals because DOs could not gain entrance to allopathic hospitals.
4. The possible positive effect of the increasing number of female doctors, both MD and DO.

PART TWO

Early Practice . . . and Beyond

THEN, THERE WERE things that sprung up in our practices—sometimes unexpectedly. Some related to recognition or acceptance and some did not. But they were attention-getting and interesting. And the tales were impressive enough to be remembered years afterward.

Tale 1

What Practice Was Like

It's good to know, as a point of reference, what practice and living were like on going into practice in the 1940s. So this Tale serves two purposes: it will let the younger readers get an idea of what faced the practitioner starting out in those early years, and it will serve as nostalgia for the generation that lived it.

Almost a century ago—there were "doctors" and "specialists." "Doctors" took care of the medical needs of the people in the community; they practiced in home-offices in neighborhoods, dispensed the best medical care of the day (and organized and coordinated the patient's medical needs), served as broad-ranged advisors to the patients on everything from health to marital counseling—and even at times on more mundane things; along with all that, they also dispensed caring, compassion, friendship, availability and many other human and humane helps. At that time, many doctors lived in the house that held their offices and it was not unusual for a neighbor-patient to knock on the doctor's door after hours because of an illness. "Specialists" were "doctors" who developed special interests in a limited area of medicine (often without formal training) and desired to spend more and more time with their new field.

Around the time I went intro practice (the late 1940s), the "doctors" had become "general practitioners." The "specialists" had started to expand and there began to spring up a sprinkling of sub-specialists. And the ratio of "doctors" to "specialists" increased with a larger percentage of specialists than before.

Practice was not the more rigid discipline that exists today. The "doctors" held "office hours." That meant they were in the office to see whatever patients came in—no appointments. So on a given day, during office hours a doctor could see seven patients (and they may have all entered the waiting room at about the same time, and had to wait their turn). The next day there might be thirty patients sitting in the waiting room. It varied, at least at the beginning, from day-to-day.

Of course, some doctors worked by appointment, but a large number depended on "walk-ins." Most specialists, who depended on referrals, maintained an appointment schedule.

It was not unusual for general practitioners to provide hospital care for some of their own office patients (depending on diagnosis). The specialists took care of patients in their specialty field (e.g., internal medicine, surgery) or consulted with the general practitioners when requested.

Therapies were much limited at the time I entered practice. Sulfonamides came into being around 1943 or so, and the first penicillin (aqueous injectable only, no oral forms) a year or two later. The Romanowski formula of long-acting penicillin was just being introduced. Anti-infection medications were miniscule compared to today's list of antibiotics in multiple forms, so we had very little to fight infections. No wonder that pediatrics practice in the early days was primarily the treatment of infectious diseases.

Talking about what medications we had then, the PDR in 1947 was a "massive" 380 pages. Now it runs more than 3,500 pages and contains listings for more than 25,000 medications.

The usual fee in the 40's for an office visit was $2—but remember economics and dollar-values were much different in those days. Then there was that other thing we did: house calls.

When a patient was too sick to come to the physician's office but not sick enough for hospitalization, we took our little black bag, loaded it with stethoscope, diagnostic set, sphygmomanometer, thermometer and perhaps a couple of other aids. Then we put in some anticipated medications; there were so few of them in those days. Off we went to the patient's home, many times traveling long distances. It was not unusual for me to make trips across the entire city of Philadelphia to make a house call.

And for this extra service, bringing the doctor's office to the patient's home, the total fee was usually $3. The startling part is that mostly we were glad to do it—that extra dollar six or eight times a week put extra food on the table. As a comparable example, my father managed a large wholesale sales force. His salesmen were happy to get the $22.50 weekly salary (notice the pennies in the salary) and were overjoyed when they earned another $5 or so each week in commissions.

Balancing all this "inexpensive" stuff, tuition for my undergraduate education at Temple University was a mere $200 a year. When I got to PCOM, the annual fee was $400 a year (and my father could not put that much together at one time for either tuition).

Most office patients paid (their parents did) at the time of service, but as I did a lot of referred hospital work (newborns, premature infants, consultations and in-patient referrals), these were billed and there was the matter of collectables; patient health insurance was not known at that time. On average, our loss on such billings was about 20-25%. At that time, many of the osteopathic hospitals (mostly small) required each physician, for support of the hospital, to pay 10% of all billings (collected or not!). So that was another loss of income. Times were different.

Some years later, the "general practitioners" (both MD and DO) became, for some reason unknown to me, officially called "family practitioners" or "family doctors" while the specialty cadre (in both professions) grew in size and expanded into more and more subspecialties.

How was life different? Let me list a few standard prices from 1946:

Coca-Cola (the original bottle)	5 cents
Hershey bar (a good size)	5 cents
Hamburger (fast food)	15 cents
Steak dinner	\$2.50-\$3.00
Daily newspaper	3 cents
Postage—letter	2 cents
Average new middle-class home	\$4,500
Average new car	\$ 1,200

Gasoline was 15 cents a gallon and the average annual wage was \$2,400. But what was life like at that time? Here is a snapshot:

Television was just starting. There were only 8 or 9 stations (for the entire United States), and no tapes or disks

There were no credit cards

There were no computers

Some outdoor plumbing could still be found

Airplanes (commercial) were two-motor jobs, and jets had not yet been invented

Automobile heaters were just starting to come into vogue, and, of course, there was no air conditioning for cars (and very little for homes)

There were no cell phones (only on Dick Tracy's wrist in the comics)

It was into this milieu that we set about practicing medicine.

TALE 2

Malpractice Insurance

THERE WAS ONE place where no distinction was made between osteopathic physicians and allopathic physicians: insurance.

Shortly after I started practice, one of the senior hospital staff members stopped me and asked, "Did you get your malpractice insurance yet?" (This was 1946).

"What?"

"Your malpractice insurance."

(For the uninitiated: at that period, little was known about, or talked about, malpractice—and litigation with massive awards was still in the future.)

"What in the world is malpractice insurance?" I asked.

With some patience (and I suspect a little glee), he answered, "It's insurance against lawsuits. Patients sometimes sue doctors for poor care, or bad results—that's what malpractice is."

"But I'm not going to do anything bad, so I don't have to worry," I said innocently.

"That's true, but sometimes these things do happen, and having insurance will pay any verdicts against you—and it can run into money. Anyway, you need it"

Struck a little scared, I asked, "But where do I get this—what you call it—malpractice insurance?"

"Any insurance broker. Do you have one?"

"No, but I'll look for one."

So I looked in the telephone book and searched around. I found an insurance broker in a corner store—he sold life insurance, casualty insurance, auto insurance—any kind, and apparently malpractice insurance was a minor part of his business.

I asked how much coverage I needed, realizing of course that as a broker he would be apt to go on the high side.

He replied, "You, know, verdicts go very high these days, so I'd suggest $50,000 worth of coverage. That would cover almost all exigencies"

Cautiously, I asked, "How much will that cost me?"

"The annual premium is $25."

At that early date in my practice, that was a lot of money. And no way could I conceive of any patient being awarded that much money for a mistake in practice, but I agreed and the transaction was completed. I had $50,000 worth of malpractice insurance for the princely sum of $25.

Little did I know, or did the broker know, nor did the senior staff member who recommended it know that by the end of the century, premiums for the most vulnerable physicians would be in the thousands, with liability coverage in the millions—and in some selected cases perhaps over a million dollars premium and ten or more million dollars coverage.

But both DOs and MDs had equality here.

Tale 3

Before 911

When I went into practice in 1946, and for years after that, there was no 911—and no rescue squads. For allopathic physicians. Or for osteopathic physicians. Or for anyone. Emergency services and trained EMTs just didn't exist, as they do today with 911 services.

So what did we do with an "emergency" on a patient who needed to be hospitalized immediately? We did it the slow way. These patients were generally ill at home; we saw them on a house call and decided that urgent hospitalization was needed—for stat oxygen or immediate surgery, or the like. Either the family found a way to bundle the patient into the family car (mostly without heat) or send for an ambulance, which meant a 30-60 minute wait and which carried none of the skilled personnel or equipment of today.

I remember specific cases—even some family members—who suffered this kind of delay. And I don't ever recall seeing any statistics on how many patients died because of the delays in getting treatment. It was the norm.

So urgent transportation was a universal problem.

But there was an added discrimination for the osteopathic physician—unintended, but circumstantial.

Family doctors (MDs), practicing in a house in a residential neighborhood, were usually the first ones who saw these urgent patients. Almost all had a connection with a neighborhood hospital or community hospital—and there were hundreds of such institutions, located in many, many neighborhoods, especially in cities and towns. So, in most instances, the trip to the hospital was rather short, and often the hospital had a connection with a community ambulance service, so the time to get to the patient's home was shorter with much time saved. And the local MD (called general practitioner in those days) either cared for the patient in that local hospital or referred the patient to a specialist, who returned that person to the local MD on discharge.

DO family physicians usually were disadvantaged. Many areas did not have an osteopathic hospital. When osteopathic hospitals, then just starting to develop, were available, there was only one (rarely two) in a town or city, meaning that for many DOs that institution was a great distance away. Frequently it was in a neighboring town—and often miles and miles from the doctor's practice area. So, the usual dilemma in emergency or urgent cases was whether to "dump" the patient in the nearest allopathic hospital for the patient's good, with non-medical consequences—acceptance of the patient by the allopathic hospital but accompanied by egregious comments about "the osteopath", often meaning loss of the patient (and his family) because the hospital referred the patient on discharge to a local MD. In much fewer situations, acceptance of their patient and return of the patient to the DO on discharge did occur.

The osteopathic physician's other alternative, and usually his preference, was to refer the patient to the osteopathic hospital across town or nearby, even though there was a longer time to get to adequate facilities. Sometimes, it was a chance of "losing the patient" either way—by death or by "patient stealing". Most DOs, of course, chose to do what was best for the patient in each case.

In some fortunate situations, a DO developed relations with specialists nearby who would treat the patient and return him or her to the DO. And in a very few cases, the emergency room would take the patient without bias. It is important to note that emergency rooms (now called emergency departments) in those days were simple and elemental, not the sophisticated treatment centers we have today.

So, while not an imposed discrimination, geography and the distant location of the DO hospital (if there was one at all) created a practice stumbling block for the osteopathic physicians.

Much of this problem is gone today, with the availability of the fantastic and ubiquitous rescue squads and the acceptance of DOs at almost every allopathic hospital—either actually on the staff or accepted as equals.

Tale 4

"Unethical" Behavior

Morton Terry, DO, was a classmate of mine at PCOM, and we were very good friends. When he finished his internal medicine residency, he moved to Miami, Florida, to practice. And practice he did—very successfully.

But a driving force in his life was his desire to set up a major osteopathic teaching institution and, eventually, an osteopathic college in Florida. (He ultimately did both—Osteopathic General Hospital and Southeastern College of Osteopathic Medicine—and served as president of both.)

Mort was a very competent internist. But early in his career, he encountered a patient with whom he felt he needed some outside help. At that time, Florida MDs did not consult with DOs, or even enter a DO hospital. And Mort's patient was in his osteopathic hospital.

However, Mort was able to snag a fine MD internist, who visited Mort's patient and consulted with Mort. Satisfactory conclusion.

Not really! The real conclusion was not so satisfactory. A day after his friend saw the patient, the MD received a telephone call from an official of the Dade County Medical Society. He was told firmly but politely that it was unethical to consult with a DO, and that he had violated an ethical rule of the Society. At the same time, he was put on notice that if it ever happened again, he would be cited for unethical conduct. Obviously, it was not considered unethical for an MD to refuse to see a patient thus allowing a patient to suffer unduly.

That was the atmosphere in the early1950s.

Interestingly, that has all disappeared. Today, the Dade County Medical Society (and Florida Medical Association) work in concert with the osteopathic profession and even solicit DOs for membership in their organizations. Similar actions are taking place all over the country today.

TALE 5

"Hello, Mort . . ."

WHEN IT FIRST came into being, Mort became interested in Nuclear Medicine. He even went to Oak Ridge and took the official U.S. government-sponsored introductory course in the field.

Then, one day a couple of years later, he noticed an advertisement for an advanced course being given at Mt. Sinai Hospital, recognized as the local "Jewish" hospital. He obtained an application and submitted it.

Shortly thereafter, he received a telephone call from the director of the course.

"Hello, Dr. Terry, we received your application. Dr. Terry, you understand that we cannot accept you because you are a DO and this course is open only to MDs. You see, Dr. Terry, we don't want any of our plans upset, so, Dr. Terry, we would like you to withdraw your application."

What Dr. Terry said is unknown but he didn't withdraw his application.

Instead, he called an official of the United Jewish Appeal, and explained the situation. He then added that since the hospital was in part aided by or subsidized by UJA, he was going to withdraw his UJA pledge and . . . it . . . was . . . a . . . sizable . . . pledge.

The next day, the director of the course called him again. "Hello, Mort" (notice that now it was Mort, not Dr. Terry) "we've been thinking it over and we are accepting your application and are going to allow you to attend the course. Mort, we will be happy to have you."

Mort delighted in telling this osteopathic tale and I am sure that years later he was delighted that Mt. Sinai now recognized and accepted osteopathic physicians, had DOs on its staff and trained DO residents.

TALE 6

Gaining a Foothold

MANY PHYSICIANS IN those days took on outside activities, generally for added income, or for a stab at professional advancement.

At a point in my early practice, I became a part-time school physician. That was an interesting aspect of pediatric medicine. It paid me a salary (that's in addition to my practice earnings) and I hoped it would expose me to more potential pediatric patients—certainly never consciously deciding to advance the osteopathic profession.

I really went into this blindly, but it suddenly struck me that as a DO, I was fully accepted by the Philadelphia School Board's Director of Health (Marie E. Frey, MD), by all the educational people and by my MD co-workers. Never did I hear a word of discrimination or even a suspicion of discrimination. In fact, a few years later, my colleague William Post,

DO, was elevated to be a district supervisor for the Medical Department.

Subsequently, more and more DOs were accepted as Philadelphia school physicians, with full acceptance and equity.

Then, as I became more and more interested in children's school health, I realized that there might be some benefit to becoming a member of the American Public Health Association, which even had a special section for school health—and I would receive their journal. I knew no one in the group and I saw no DO names, but (I guess being a brash youth) I applied anyway, and was accepted. Sometime after becoming a member of APHA, I was told that I was the first DO to join the group. Of course, I was proud. And then, a few years later, I applied to become a Fellow of the APHA, not knowing what qualifications or restrictions there were. Lo and behold, I made it! and became the first DO FAPHA.

I was doubly proud—I felt it advanced my career, plus gave me much personal learning and satisfaction. It never entered my thoughts as creating an advance for osteopathic medicine (it was "osteopathy" in those days). But, in retrospect, that plus similar actions of many other DOs across the country, created new steps in that direction: 1, plus 1, plus 1, plus 1, equals . . . well, you know.

TALE 7

The White House Conferences

SINCE 1909, AND every ten years, some sort of federal conference was held in Washington on considerations of children's health, all White House sponsored.

But the really big one came in 1960, under the direction of President Dwight D. Eisenhower. It was the 1960 White House Conference on Children and Youth and it actually celebrated the golden anniversary of White House conferences. President Eisenhower himself addressed the Conference.

At first, there did not seem to be invitations for osteopathic physicians at this 1960 meeting (none attended previous conferences). But, somehow, the AOA and the American College of Osteopathic Pediatricians were allowed delegates. I can't recall whether the AOA or the ACOP initiated it—but we were there. And it doesn't matter who deserved or got the credit—both participated.

That conference had 7,000 delegates and the size necessitated formation of 210 different work groups. The osteopathic delegates were the six DOs: Myron Magen, DO, Frank Souders, DO, Virginia Poole Ellis, DO, Leo C. Wagner, DO, Kenneth Mahoney, DO, and Arnold Melnick, DO. All were Fellows of the ACOP.

There were full and plentiful programs on children and it went on for a full week, with all the color, display, and hoopla accompanying it, ala Washington. Interesting, enjoyable and educational, maybe because there was widespread participation—physicians, educators, social workers, psychologists, just to name a few. And perhaps that was part of the reason for including DOs—to give a well-rounded consideration to the problems of children in 1960.

I do not remember any world-shattering conclusions or promises coming out of it, or out of the follow-ups. Perhaps the greatest product of the Conference was the formation of the National Committee on Children and Youth, formed to advance understanding and care of American children. But it was a landmark (of which we could be proud and could brag). It gave each of the participants a wide view on the total situation. And for us, the DO delegates, it meant hobnobbing with multiple professions and mixing (as DOs) with some of them on an individual basis, while at the same time learning. At least, we could say that the osteopathic profession was accepted, even if it weren't an "official recognition".

I am sure the same thing happened to the other delegates, but on return hone, I was appointed to a couple of Pennsylvania and Philadelphia child health committees. Perhaps it was minor and personal recognition, but in its small way, added to the acceptance of the osteopathic profession.

In 1970, another ten-year Conference was held—and again with osteopathic representation. From then on, the WHCs seemed to fizzle away.

But we were there! And it was another step forward.

Tale 8

And Another Step

It's amazing how much serendipity and chance encounters modify our lives. Early in my practice years (1958), I joined the American Medical Writers Association, a sort of small coterie of people interested in medical writing (about 400 members then, about 5000 now). I signed on because of my similar interests.

Interesting sidelight (in view of our discussion on MD discrimination): AMWA was originally a very small group of MDs and the criterion for membership was an MD degree. After some years of existence, they allowed non-MDs to join. When they created the Fellow degree for AMWA, it was limited to MDs only. That persisted for many years, and then it was rescinded. Thereupon, two PhDs became president, and a couple of years later, I was elected to that office (after serving as president of the Delaware Valley Chapter).

I was the first (and only) DO president—in its 34th year—1975.

One of the friends I made in this organization was one George Stickley, an editor for Lippincott, who subsequently went into the publishing business as George F. Stickley Company. Not long after that, I completed the manuscript for my first book and, fearing another DO rejection from a "standard" publisher, took it to George. He liked the book but explained why he could not undertake it. But he referred me to Warren Green, a personal friend of his and an established medical publisher—with his recommendation. Warren published the book.

While it set no records, *Pediatrics: Some Uncommon Views on Some Common Problems* did make the print list (in 1975)—one of the first tomes authored by a DO in a specialty field. It became one of the early beachheads (more like a grain of sand) in the publishing side of osteopathic medicine.

Another step forward—like so many of my colleagues were doing at the same time in their fields of interest.

PART THREE

The Merger

IN 1961—JUST AS there were small steps being gained in the recognition of osteopathic medicine—there occurred in California a momentous event: the California Osteopathic Association merged with the California Medical Association, taking with it the College of Osteopathic Physicians and Surgeons and the only publicly-supported osteopathic hospital in the country—the osteopathic branch of the Los Angeles County Hospital.

Opinions on this "merger" vary widely but it shook the osteopathic profession outside of California, and is still remembered as a significant event in osteopathic history.

Tale 1

A Look at the "Merger"

I write this as a surviving witness to the times and some scenes of the "merger". For years on either side of the "merger", I was active politically in AOA and the Pennsylvania Osteopathic Association. In 1959-1960, I was President of the POA and I sat as a Pennsylvania delegate to the AOA House of Delegates for several years, including 1961, the year of the "merger". That was over 50 years ago and memory of specific details may not always be accurate after that length of time, but the actual story is correct.

California, the first state to grant DOs unlimited licenses (1901) was one of the fastest growing states in the osteopathic profession. In 1961, they were the largest state in osteopathic membership, over 2500. In part because of their size and their forward-looking activities and accomplishments, they were a powerhouse osteopathically. They had the largest delegation in the

House, where they wielded strong influence, and were also extremely powerful in the Board of Trustees.

For many years, the Los Angeles County Hospital had devoted a special area as an osteopathic unit. Around 1958, by a public plebiscite in the county, a new and separate osteopathic unit was built; it was operated by DOs, perhaps the only such osteopathic publicly-supported hospital at that time. California carried much weight in AOA politics and activities, they knew it and they used it. Being a political powerhouse, California was often at odds with the rest of the AOA House of Delegates.

There had been rumors in the fifties (or earlier) of talks about California somehow combining with the allopathic group. The interplay between the California Osteopathic Association and the California Medical Association became known in the fall of 1961; it was rumored that underground merger papers had been created. At the AOA House of Delegates, California introduced a motion relating to the potential merger, and when it was totally rejected by the House, the entire California delegation, as a unit (and probably on a signal from their leaders), rose and walked out of the House—never to return.

Subsequently, we found out that the merger included:

1. Handing over the College of Osteopathic Medicine and Surgery (for $1) to the CMA for conversion to an allopathic school. It was later

moved and re-christened as the Cal State-Irvine Medical School.

2. Allowing DOs to secure an MD degree for $65, and then request the California Board of Osteopathic Examiners for a transfer to the California Medical Board.
3. Turning over control of the osteopathic unit of L.A. County Hospital to CMA.
4. Funds controlled by the COA were to be utilized, in part, to obtain public approval of the necessary changes in the Osteopathic Act of 1922 to approve the merger.

Then by another public vote, the licensing of any additional DOs in California was prohibited, thus essentially ending the existence of osteopathic medicine in California.

TALE 2

. . . and the Sequelae

FIRST, IT SHOULD be noted that not all DOs in California felt overwhelming approval of the "merger". Feelings varied from complete approval to complete rejection. In the latter category, about 200 osteopathic physicians rejected the call and refused to apply for the MD degree. Among those who applied, I felt there were three general groups: those who were enthusiastic (or at least satisfied); those who were sort of indifferent to it but followed the crowd (or hoped it would fend off any possible losses from the "merger"); and those who applied but were not really happy with it, but found it expedient.

To loyalists in California and the rest of the country, it seemed as if the CMA were trying to eliminate the osteopathic profession, and many suspected that the AMA was participating behind the scenes. There occurred no rush of DOs from around the country to get into California and get an MD degree. On the contrary, as soon as the revived Osteopathic Board of Examiners was established years later, about 125 DOs took the initial examination for a DO license (1974).

As for the motives of the pro-merger DOs, Ethan Allen (1) said it succinctly, "I think they were more interested in the prestige in the community . . . They felt that they would have more prestige if they had MD after their name."

In addition to the 200-some California DOs who did not apply for the new degree, as early as 1961 there began a resurgence among the loyalists to revive the osteopathic profession. With DO leaders like Drs. Allen, Richard Eby, Edna Lay and others, the group that wanted to maintain the osteopathic profession quickly organized the Osteopathic Physicians and Surgeons of California. What they started led to two major developments:

> One of their earliest actions was devoted to re-installing the right of DOs to practice in California. They sued the state on "civil rights" grounds in a class action. Although losing on the first legal round, in 1974 the California Supreme Court reversed itself and the DOs won, establishing the right of DOs to be licensed and practice again.

> OPSC flourished and grew and attracted more and more osteopathic physicians. Today, California is the third largest osteopathic state with more than 5400 DOs. Plus, along with that progress, two new osteopathic colleges were developed and are operating most successfully.

Once the merger was completed, the COA assigned all former DOs to a single district society, regardless of where they lived or practiced—the 41st Medical Trust. This move kept all former-osteopathic voters (and votes) to a small fraction of the total CMA voters—and thus limited any possible power or influence of the "new-MDs".

TALE 3

Effect on Osteopathic Progress

EXCEPT FOR ONE group, the "merger" provided no *quid pro quo* or direct benefit to any DOs. The merger-ites immediately gained all the recognition and benefits accorded MDs.

I and others believe that the "merger" brouhaha stimulated some considerations: Did it impact the great progress of the osteopathic profession throughout the United State—either enhancing it or retarding it? Perrotta (2) summed it up nicely with the feelings of the Chicago College student body (at that time) which "was convinced that either the end of the osteopathic medical profession was near and our school would close or, alternatively, that our school would soon be granting the 'little MD degree'"

That was the dilemma of most osteopathic physicians at that time—and there were DOs on both sides of the question. But, by and large, I believe that the majority of DOs felt, as Perrotta later (2) said, ". . . imbued with a sense of purpose, resolve, pride, and dignity, which gave them the vision, fortitude, and perseverance to survive . . ." My own belief is that, consciously or unconsciously, it made most of us strive just a little harder to achieve equality and acceptance.

While I am not giving this event credit for what the profession has accomplished over the years, I do think it was another small step—like other tales in this book and combining with them—leading to the present day acceptance and recognition, which is almost universal.

My observation is that, today, there are fewer cries for us to embrace the MD degree and more feelings of satisfaction with the progress that has brought us—as DOs—to a point of near-equality. We have won all the many advantages that physicians should have and never had to give up our birthright to get them!

REFERENCES

1. *Interview with Ethan Allen, DO, FACOFP.* Archival & Historical Committee, ACOFP, 2007
2. Perrotta AL: *Whatever you are, be a good one* (letter) J Am Osteopath Assoc. 111(9), 2011, pp. 528-528.
3. Melnick, A: *Whatever you are, be a good one* (letter). J Am Osteopath Assoc 111(9), 2011, pp. 529-530

PART FOUR

The CHOP Years

CHOP is Children's Hospital of Philadelphia, always an outstanding institution and an epitome of excellent child care. A lot of my experiences in practice were related to CHOP. At first, I had "connections" with CHOP, that is, I knew a few physicians there, sent very occasional cases there and felt comfortable, but I had no official affiliation. Later in my practice years, as you will see, I had an official connection. I spent an infinitesimal amount of time at CHOP compared to my primary practice—two private offices and two osteopathic hospitals at which I was Chairman of the Department of Pediatrics and where I admitted all my patients. The only measurable time I spent at CHOP was in my final three years there when I volunteered one day a week for a couple of hours in the Adolescent Clinic. But my connection was an influential and important part of my life because, in retrospect, this era represents an analogy to the gradually increasing acceptance of osteopathic physicians by the allopathic branch of the healing arts.

TALE 1

A Look Back

TO UNDERSTAND MY CHOP years, I must take the reader back a few years, perhaps 1942-44.

CHOP had always had a highly-regarded Friday Clinical Conference, held weekly and featuring interesting and important in-house cases, with intense discussion from one or more Attending Staff members. It was a great learning experience. In addition to residents, medical students and CHOP staff members, many community pediatricians attended either regularly or on a sporadic basis. So it was not unusual to find strange faces in the audience.

Leo Wagner, DO, was one of the leading osteopathic pediatricians in the Philadelphia area, an attending at Osteopathic Hospital of Philadelphia and highly regarded for his skills and competence. I am not sure whether this incident took place the first time he attended the Conference or after he had attended several.

But, on one Friday (before I interned), he went into the CHOP auditorium, and took a seat. Shortly, the physician-in-chief of CHOP approached him, and said, "Sir, I'll have to ask you to leave. This conference is only for pediatricians." Dr. Wagner replied, "But I am a pediatrician. I'm an osteopathic pediatrician." The final blow came with the answer, "But this is only for MDs. You'll have to leave."

Dr. Wagner left, never to return. One may wonder why this happened. There were no medical secrets, not even trade secrets—only good, clear medical information. Cynics might question whether they were afraid someone would learn something—something that might eventually help patients. There is (and was) no logical explanation except that, in that era, MDs did not accept DOs as physicians or as any part of the health care team.

That was the 40's atmosphere.

Tale 2

How It Could Happen

Readers may wonder how Dr. Wagner was singled out—or recognized in this open conference. Thereby hangs another tale of professional discrimination, and a sort of personally painful one.

F. Munro (Jim) Purse, DO, also a respected osteopathic faculty pediatrician and one of my professors, was a regular attendee at these meetings for quite a while—undetected—and even became friendly with several other regulars—without becoming identified as a DO (something we often hid in those days in such circumstances). One of those regulars was my uncle, an MD.

Very soon after I finished my internship, I grasped at the opportunity to attend these sessions and advance my knowledge. So I went.

At one session, I saw my uncle shortly after I entered the auditorium and I waved to him. Jim was sitting next to him. My uncle leaned over to Jim and whispered, "I wonder if they know who's here in the audience." Surprised at the remark, Jim asked, "Who's here?" My uncle replied, "I see an osteopath sitting over there," referring to me. No empathy, just inbred discrimination.

Fortunately, he apparently did not mention it to anyone else and fortunately I was never asked to leave the Friday Conference, but this tale shows that discrimination, as it always does, crosses all relationship lines, even family. Eventually, I attended as many as I could get to, undetected first and later accepted,.

There was one situation that puzzled me, but I understood it. While DOs (just a few) were fighting and struggling (and sort of "sneaking" in) to obtain just a little more knowledge to help their patients, some allopathic medical students sat in the back of the room at the Clinical Conferences—reading newspapers or magazines.

Tale 3

On the Other Hand . . .

But there were exceptions to the discrimination. One outstanding one was Irving J. Wolman, MD. My first contact with Dr. Wolman was shortly before he became chief of pediatric pathology and attending physician at CHOP.

Here's how I met him. I had written an original article, in my internship days, about the blood counts of newborns: *An Index for Children's Blood Counts*. It was published in the Journal of the American Osteopathic Association. Julian Mines, DO, an obstetrician at Osteopathic Hospital and one of my teachers, had already had several original articles published, and he gave me some sage advice. He suggested that since the work was original, I should pick out 5 or 6 outstanding MD pediatricians and 5 or 6 leading MD hematologists and send a copy of the article to each of them and ask for comments or criticisms; he sort of told me what to expect—some no replies, some hostile comments and maybe a few helpful suggestions.

One of those I selected (blindly) was Dr. Wolman, a pediatric hematologist, then at St. Christopher's Hospital for Children in Philadelphia. At that time, I did not know him or that he was certified in four specialties.

About two weeks after sending the reprints, late one night as I was going upstairs to bed, my telephone rang. Dr. Wolman identified himself and apologized for the late call. "I just finished reading your article." he said, "and I would like you to come down to St. Chris and discuss it with me."

At that point, I would have gone to visit him at midnight—to get even this little recognition from an accredited MD, but I made an appointment to meet him at his hospital a couple of days later.

When I arrived, his secretary told me that he was busy in his laboratory, but directed me to go into his office and wait for him. While I was sitting there, a resident came in. We said a quick hello and he went about his work. A few minutes later, Dr. Wolman arrived, we shook hands and he said to the resident, "Did you meet Dr. Melnick?" He said that he had not and then asked of me, "Where are you from?" Detecting a note of looking-down-his-nose waiting to tell of his prestigious medical school (as I later realized), Dr. Wolman immediately interrupted, "Dr. Melnick is from the Osteopathic Hospital. Did you read his article on my desk? If not, I want you to read it and tell me why you didn't think of it."

We went on to discuss my article, and thus began a long and beautiful friendship and, as I did not realize then, another step in improving allopathic-osteopathic relations.

Dr. Wolman did not care that I was a DO. Dr. Wolman did not care that my article was published in an osteopathic journal. Dr. Wolman cared only about Pediatrics and those who contributed—or potentially contributed—to the field.

He bore no discriminatory feelings.

Not long after that, Dr. Wolman—now Irv—transferred to CHOP and our deep friendship continued and ripened. So he is an important part of my CHOP tales.

Tale 4

Profiting from Contacts

Irv Wolman, now being a personal friend, also served as a point man for me in developing new contacts at CHOP. Over the years, I made many additional contacts. And that served an immediate purpose—plus a delayed one.

I was active in osteopathic organizational affairs. At times, I served as Program Chairman or President of the Eastern Association of Osteopathic Pediatricians (mostly Philadelphia and vicinity) and the American College of Osteopathic Pediatricians. I had occasions to seek speakers for our pediatric meetings and I called on a number of people from CHOP, many through the help of Dr. Wolman It was a valuable source of pediatric lecturers and, even though I did not recognize it at the time, a burgeoning cog in the wheel of acceptance and recognition of my profession—actually my branch (osteopathic) of the medical profession.

One of those contacts was C. Everett ("Chick") Koop, MD, world famous pediatric surgeon and chief at CHOP. I had a few occasions—not many—to utilize his great services for patients too complicated for my surgeon-colleagues (DOs). And I used him for several programs (he was also an outstanding lecturer).

"Chick" became a personal friend. He had some remarkable philosophies of practice—all benefiting the patients. Once I heard that he had made a house-call on the family of a child who had died at CHOP. Questioned on it, he strongly explained that a doctor's work is not over when a patient dies; he felt that a physician has some responsibility to the family of that child to help ease their grief. What a heart!

Perhaps the outstanding evidence of his character was the decision he made when appointed Surgeon-General of the United States. He faced a few conflicts because of some strongly-held personal beliefs. Putting them aside, he essentially said, "It's no longer my beliefs that count. I am now the nation's physician and I must consider everyone." And he did just that!

He remained a friend until he died and I am so privileged and proud that he wrote the Foreword to my book *Professionally Speaking: Public Speaking for Health Professionals (1998)*.

And each of these contacts and each of these speakers further spread the word of Osteopathic Medicine. In a word, I think that a few of them learned that "osteopaths" did not have horns. A victory!

Tale 5

An Invitation to Be First

One afternoon, I was sitting in Irv Wolman's office, chatting about a number of things, when in the course of chewing over multiple topics, I casually mentioned that I and my partner (Robert Berger, DO) had been seeing a number of children referred to us to be hospitalized for toxicity from the administration of Compazine (prophenothiazine) to control nausea and vomiting.

Irv seemed to perk up with this bit of information and he started asking questions. Then he said, "This has not yet been reported in the literature. How about collecting the data and doing an article for Clinical Pediatrics?" Irv had been editor of that journal since its inception, and he apparently thought this was worthwhile. Up to that point I had not considered publishing that material.

So we did as he asked and submitted the article which was published—*Phenothiazine Reactions in Children* (1967). Until the article came out, we did not realize that this would be the first DO-authored article ever published in Clinical Pediatrics and maybe one of the first in any allopathic Pediatrics journal—a first for us—and another step in the right direction for the profession.

Subsequently, we published other articles in Clinical Pediatrics. Then, one day, Irv said to me, "Arnold, I want to appoint you to the Editorial Board of Clinical Pediatrics." I thanked him profusely, realizing that this was the first time a DO would be appointed to the Editorial Board of an allopathic publication. And appoint me, he did. The following month, my name and my degree—Arnold Melnick, DO—appeared on the masthead, along with all the MD members of the Editorial Board. I was—and am—very proud. The masthead continued that way for another issue or two and then, WOW! Suddenly the masthead dropped all degrees—MD as well as my DO degree; all Board members were listed simply as "Dr." with no degree.

I never found out why that happened. I can postulate several discriminatory reasons but I don't know. I do know that it was not Irv's idea and that he did not approve of it, but there was obviously no rational reason for it.

So that one afternoon's discussion led to two firsts for me—and another step in the acceptance of osteopathic physicians.

Tale 6

Another Invitation and Progress

This tale is yet another instance of Irv Wolman's refusal to be included in the ranks of those practicing discrimination.

As I did every so often, I took some blood slides to Irv for interpretation—slides from a child who had puzzling presentations. I went to his office and his secretary explained that he was not in the office because he was tied up conducting a three-day course at CHOP on Pediatric Hematology. Somehow, I got to see him and his first reaction was to say, "Arnold, why don't you come down and sit in on the course?"

In part, I was embarrassed by the invitation. I had seen the course advertised (for a fee) and, after considering the fact that as a DO I would not be accepted, I decided not to try to register for it. Now I was being invited to sit in (without a fee). I explained to Irv my original dilemma and explained that I did not want to embarrass him by submitting an application. Irv's immediate response. "I'm inviting you to sit in for the remaining two days of the course. If they don't want to take your money, that's their problem. I'm inviting you."

Once again, his interest was in Pediatrics, those who would contribute to it or benefit from it. And he was willing to let anybody learn—whether DO or MD.

Discrimination was not in Irving Wolman's vocabulary—one of a growing number of cooperative MDs who were going out of their way to work with DOs. And it certainly helped us.

TALE 7

An Invitation I Couldn't Refuse

AL BONGIOVANNI, MD, was a celebrated pediatric endocrinologist at CHOP, widely noted for his research. He was also a fine individual, free of prejudice—and ultimately a friend of mine. (Actually, we learned later, and it had no influence on our relationship that his father and my father had been acquaintances in their earlier lives.).

When the position of physician-in-chief opened—about three-quarters of the way through my CHOP experience—Al was appointed to the post. Not long after that, he contacted me; I don't remember the time or circumstance but he said he wanted to see me.

After greeting me, Al said, "Arnold, I want you to apply for our staff." How flattering! There were no DOs on the CHOP staff and he was asking me to apply. I was quick to say to him, "Al, you know as well as I the differences between MDs and DOs and you know all the problems with interrelationships. So, I think it better if I do not apply—and I seriously am flattered—but just allow me to continue the same fine relationship I have with you and so many staff members and with the hospital. Thanks, but no thanks."

Immediately, he responded, "'Chick' Koop and I talked it over and we both want you on the staff." Chick was Chairman of the Surgical Staff and Al was Chairman of the Medical Staff.

Still somewhat reluctant, but thrilled, I did apply and ultimately I became the first DO on the CHOP staff. This was a high-point in my professional life, but it wasn't the end. It carried with it a faculty appointment at the University of Pennsylvania School of Medicine, another serendipitous "first".

Interestingly, months later, I attended a seminar in Trenton, NJ, and at the luncheon, I was seated next to a physician I did not know. After some small talk, I learned that he had previously been connected with the Dean's Office at Penn. I mentioned that I was connected with CHOP. Then, he asked me my name. I told him "Melnick".

"Of course, I know your name." he said. "You know that in order to be appointed to the staff at CHOP, one must have a Penn faculty appointment. So when your name came to the Dean's Office (as added to the CHOP staff), we spent about three months debating whether we should include a DO on the Penn faculty—we never had a DO on the faculty before. In the end, we decided it was satisfactory and we approved your faculty position and your CHOP staff membership."

Thus, in one operation, I achieved two firsts: First DO as a CHOP staff member and first DO on Penn faculty. But, in the long run, I believe its importance was that it was another step forward for the osteopathic profession, and wider acceptance for DOs, a foot-in-the-door if you will—and at a prestigious allopathic institution.

Tale 8

Those Remnant "Oh"s

While the acceptance and recognition of DOs continue to grow, there are always—and always will be—remnants of "discrimination".

Even after being appointed to the staff at CHOP, there were some instances in which my recognition was that of "the osteopath". Maybe it requires a large number of DOs on the staff before people start to eliminate that.

Two incidents I remember:

Once, while walking though the hospital, I ran into "Chick" Koop talking with another staff member. I stopped to say hello, and "Chick" asked the doctor "Do you know Dr. Melnick?" Pausing to think for a moment, he responded, "Ohhh . . . ohhhh . . . , yes" meaning "the osteopath."

Harold Finkel's son-in-law, Bill Moskowitz, MD, had applied for a residency after graduating from the

University of Pennsylvania School of Medicine. Lewis Barness, MD, an outstanding faculty member and a highly-regarded "rock" of the CHOP staff, had observed Bill during his school years and wrote a very strong letter of recommendation to CHOP. Hearing nothing, Harold asked me (now a new CHOP staff member) also to write a letter of recommendation, which I did. Again, nothing was heard, and I asked another prominent staff member to inquire from the Residency Director. When asked about Bill Moskowitz, the Director was puzzled . . . thought a while . . . and then said, "Oh, yes, he's the one who was recommended by the osteopath." Dr. Barness's letter was apparently secondary to him—in spite of his being a distinguished senior staff member. Discrimination dies hard. Bill was eventually accepted and was an exemplary resident. He is now a leading faculty member at another university.

I am glad this tale is short.

Tale 9

Real Progress

Progress continued—more and more acceptance.

In 1976, when I retired from private practice, I went to see David Cornfeld, MD, who had succeeded Al Bongiovanni, MD, as Physician-in-Chief of CHOP. I had met Dave and went to him with this request: I have retired from practice and would now like to give back to CHOP for all that I had received from that institution. Dave was quite cooperative. No "osteopath". No questions of degree differences. No stalling. No restrictions. Just doing the right thing.

Dave made several suggestions—offering opportunities for me. I chose to serve on the initial staff of Adolescent Medicine. Four pediatricians were involved and we operated an adolescent clinic two days a week. My role was one day a week for a couple of hours. I met no discrimination, or even intimations of it. We were colleagues, and I was treated as such by all the other pediatricians I met. I served there until I moved to Florida in 1980.

Along the way, another movement of progress occurred. One pediatrician in this group suggested forming a Philadelphia Adolescent Society and proceeded to organize it. Over the few years that I was still in Philadelphia, I served as Program Chairman, selected by the otherwise-MD membership. And no signs of discrimination.

We had come a long way—both CHOP and the osteopathic profession.

Commentary

These are a few of the tales connected with my work with Children's Hospital of Philadelphia. Strung together, they represent a sampling of the progress in recognition and acceptance that was taking place all over the United States—a microcosm of the country-wide phenomenon I am sure that many other DOs have their own tales illustrating the same climb.

Recognizing fully the fantastic work done by our osteopathic organizations with their influence and pressure, much of osteopathic medicine's growth and progress is attributable to contacts, friendships and connections created by individual DOs in their everyday work—one DO at a time, one MD at a time, all over the United States—adding up to the almost total acceptance today. And CHOP is just one example—a good one—of that.

Even though there were problems at the beginning—as there were all over the country—I am proud of and pleased with the movement at CHOP—not an organized program but a gradual recognition of the need for change. I included many CHOP tales because, in retrospect, the CHOP tales are a microcosm of the larger and more influential growth and acceptance of the osteopathic profession by the world around us

They were great years. Although it was only a small part of my professional life, CHOP contributed greatly to it, educationally as well as in recognition. And I am grateful for it.

PART FIVE

Writing and Speaking

I HAVE ALWAYS HAD a serious interest in writing and public speaking. Maybe that carried over to my professional life. For programs I was associated with, I always wanted the best possible speakers—and tried to influence that even when I was not directly responsible for it.

I never approached those two interests with the goal in mind that it would advance the osteopathic profession. But now, looking back, I realize that every instance did just that.

Maybe not world-shattering, but every step forward added to osteopathic prestige.

Tale 1

Ubiquitous Flag-wavers

A most influential but unrecognized group that aided the great progress of osteopathic medicine is one I call Ubiquitous Flag-wavers, the hundreds of DOs who, over the past 70 years in their own communities and elsewhere, have addressed probably thousands of groups all over the country on a wide variety of medical topics. You know, DOs speaking at PTA meetings, service clubs, various organizations, commercial groups, and with a total mix of audiences. Whether they set out to or not, they represented the osteopathic profession; in a positive way, they were waving our flag.

Almost none of these DOs did this specifically to aggrandize our profession; they merely wanted to inform their audiences about medical topics, as invited by the organizers of those meetings, or in some cases to comply with a patient's request to help out by speaking to a group. Sometimes speakers did this to encourage referrals in a professional way, hoping to garner more patients for their practices. Almost all of these were freebies; they did not go on the promise of compensation.

But hidden in each presentation was a special message: I am an osteopathic physician—a real doctor—and have the ability to inform patients and families about medical topics. The better the speaker (and speech), the more the hidden flag-waving occurred.

During my career, I made a number of these speeches. This is not meant to imply that because an osteopathic physician gave a talk, the audience suddenly became osteopathic converts. The mind-set of the listeners who heard these talks was almost as different as the individual hearers.

What I am convinced of is that some listeners went away with the same negative views they came with. A good talk also produced these results: some of the listeners had a small improvement in their opinions of osteopathic medicine, some felt more acceptable of osteopathic medicine and some—a very few—went away now enthusiastic. But considering the volume of these speeches over the years and across the country, osteopathic medicine profited and we moved a step closer to acceptance.

Another force moving us toward greater acceptance and recognition.

Tale 2

Atlantic Post Graduate Assembly

In the 1960s, Harold Finkel, DO, and I organized the Atlantic Post Graduate Assembly, a private enterprise, for the purpose of providing high quality osteopathic educational programs outside restrictive bounds such as timing, location and limitation of speakers. At first, our programs were provided at resort locations, and later at foreign spots, such as London and Rome. We ran for perhaps seven or eight years.

For our outside speakers, we chose those we thought were the best—without regard to being rejected or refused, neither of which ever happened. The issue of "osteopathic" never arose, even though all our letter-invitations were signed Arnold Melnick, DO. Perhaps just "guts" was the better part of valor. And we were fortunate to snare some outstanding speakers—big "names".

One of our prizes was Morris Fishbein, MD, internationally-known spokesman at one time for the AMA, and for many years the icon of medical writing. He accepted and gave a wonderful talk. I seized the opportunity to have lunch with him, for I figured this was our chance to tell him something about the osteopathic profession. To my surprise, I spent time mostly listening. Dr. Fishbein told me things that I never knew about osteopathic medicine and the profession—not complaints or other negatives, as I would have expected, but factual and non-judgmental.

But he went away having met some DOs and having heard some osteopathic lecturers and having been exposed to our quality programs. I do not know whether it changed his mind about anything (or if it needed changing), but he did get to see some positive things about us.

That was a move forward for the profession.

A number of other prominent MDs were given similar exposure not only in this organization but throughout the country

Tale 3

Other Speakers

APGA was not the only osteopathic organization that invited well-known speakers and unconsciously in the process, advanced the osteopathic image.

The Pennsylvania Osteopathic Association (now the Pennsylvania Osteopathic Medical Association), like other state osteopathic organizations, was inviting excellent non-osteopathic speakers for its educational programs.

Two that I was associated with provided interesting stories. Again, invitations were signed with the DO degree. And never did we have an objection or question.

I invited Alfred C Kinsey, ScD, at the peak of his fame for his Kinsey Report and author of *Sexual Behavior in the Human Male* (and later, *Female)* to speak at one of our conventions. He accepted tentatively but could not promise definitely. He offered to keep the date open if I would wait. I did . . . and did . . . and did. I don't know where I got the courage but I advertised his appearance and hoped. At last, just two weeks before the convention, he told me he would be there.

He delivered an engaging speech, attracting one of the largest audiences I had ever seen at a divisional society meeting.

And now I realize that he must have gone away with a positive concept of the osteopathic profession—or even more positive if he already was in our camp.

In another instance, we invited Reverend Norman Vincent Peale to deliver the keynote address. He was a renowned radio preacher and the highly-recognized author of the best-selling *The Power of Positive Thinking.* Of course, he presented a sparkling and exciting address.

Afterward, I sat with him to listen to the following speaker, the fantastic orator, Otterbein Dressler, DO, then Dean of the Philadelphia College of Osteopathy. Midway through Dr. Dressler's talk, Dr. Peale turned to me and asked, "Where did you get such a magnificent speaker?"

Did that help enhance his image of the osteopathic profession? I'm sure that whatever his previous position on osteopathic medicine, it grew. One person, one at a time, the profession advanced in acceptance and recognition.

Tale 4

Impressing the Speaker

Part of the reaction of our outside speakers to osteopathic medicine comes with how we impress them with what we are doing.

Waldo Nelson, MD, was an internationally-known pediatrician, professor at Temple University Medical School and head of St. Christopher's Hospital for Children in Philadelphia. He was even better known as the editor of *Textbook of Pediatrics,* the ultimate standard for pediatrics for many years and through multiple editions. So it was that the American College of Osteopathic Pediatricians invited him in 1988 to give the annual James M. Watson Memorial Lecture, the first non-member of ACOP ever to be thus honored.

The meeting was in San Francisco, and Dr. Nelson notified us that he would attend for the first day, having to return to Philadelphia thereafter. Following his talk, which was splendid, he stayed a couple of hours to hear some of our home-grown speakers. By the end of that first day, he postponed his return and stayed for the entire program.

Did we impress him? I sure think we did. And did that enhance his views on osteopathic physicians? I would think so. I don't think he came with any biased view because he had worked with Joseph Dieterle, DO, who was one of the first DO residents at St. Chris—and an outstanding one, too—and Robert Berger, DO, my practice partner who trained and practiced Pediatric Neurology at that hospital. (Both were past presidents of the American College of Osteopathic Pediatricians.)

But for someone so entrenched in allopathic medicine to be so impressed with an osteopathic program would almost guarantee that we gained points with him. And, with it, more growth in acceptance and approval.

Tale 5

The Writing Effect

Through our writing as osteopathic physicians, even though it may not be extensive, or world-shaking, we also influence perceptions about our profession, sometimes for good, sometimes for bad. I have already recounted my connection with Irving Wolman, MD (see Part 4, Tale 3). That came about through a published research article of mine—and the tremendous exposure that contact gave me.

I have published many articles, some of them in allopathic (or non-specific) publications. In many cases, I was the first osteopathic physician to appear in those journals. Among those are Medical Economics (at its peak of popularity), Medical Opinion, Journal of Medical Education, Academic Medicine and Science Editor, to name just a few.

Even though I claim no great attributes for any of my work, at least they were good enough to be accepted for publication and for their readers' viewing. And I am sure that among their readership were some allopathic physicians who might have taken on a new, or improved, stance on osteopathic medicine because of it.

Never did I set out to write for that specific purpose. In fact, I never even considered it. But I think that each article published by an osteopathic physician—especially in allopathic journals—has a tendency to increase the recognition and acceptance of our profession.

Today, many of our DOs have published in "MD" journals—and among them, the most prestigious ones around. No one article "advanced" the profession, but each was a positive step in the right direction.

Tale 6

Foreign Intrigue

ONE OF THE Atlantic Post Graduate Assembly's trips was to Rome. I had chosen several local speakers of prominence. During the entire stay in Rome and interaction with a number of outstanding MDs, never was the word "osteopath" mentioned or questioned, never were our credentials challenged, and never was there any display or hint of discrimination. We were accepted as physicians!

The first memorable anecdote was pure humanity.

On the opening morning, I was standing in the lobby of the hotel looking for the featured speaker, a noted Italian surgeon. A gentleman entered the hotel and walked over to me. "Are you Dr. Melnick?" he asked in English with the usual Italian-tinged accent.

I acknowledged that I was, and he continued, "I am Dr. X. Unfortunately, Dr. A is unable to be here and he asked me to substitute for him." With the program start 15 minutes away, I had little choice but to accept. Dr. X made a splendid presentation and I thanked him profusely for filling in at the last minute. And I must admit, I did have flashes of an internationally-known speaker "dumping off" the DOs to a junior member.

And my program was saved. But wait!

That afternoon, I was approached by another gentleman. He introduced himself as Dr. A, the originally-scheduled speaker. I quickly explained that Dr. X had shown up and was an admirable substitute, and I thanked him for sending him.

He put his hand up for me to stop. "No," he said, "you do not understand. I came to apologize for not being here. I had to stay at the hospital this morning because my wife was being operated on for breast cancer." What courage! What a feeling of responsibility!

Expressing my sorrow at his situation, I thanked him so much for coming to the hotel anyway. And I wondered if I could have done what he did. And it shattered any bit of suspicion I may have had.

A foreign acceptance of osteopathic medicine and a generous display of magnificent humanism—what more could I ask?

The second remembered incident was quite humorous, even though not related.

This Italian specialist who was scheduled to speak showed up with another person tagging along. When he introduced himself, also introduced the other gentleman with, "I am unsure of my ability with English, so I brought along my friend who will translate for me."

Wondering how this would work out, I (without any other recourse) agreed.

My scheduled speaker took to the podium, and even though he carried an Italian accent, he spoke beautifully and delivered an understandable and interesting paper.

Then, it was time for questions and answers. He explained to our audience that his friend would translate the questions into Italian for him, he would reply in Italian, and the interpreter would explain in English what he said.

The first question went this round-robin without difficulty. Then, the second. Then the third. The fourth questioner spoke, and the same pattern started. When the interpreter translated the Italian answer into English, the professor interrupted, "No! No! No! That's nota whata I said. I said . . ." and he proceeded to give the answer, his way, in perfect English. And the audience applauded loudly.

His English ability exceeded what he thought it was. A successful routine and a satisfied audience. And a speaker whose concern was that the group understood his point.

Not a whimper of any kind of discrimination or question about the audience's credentials.

And another small step for Osteopathic Medicine—even though in a foreign country.

PART SIX

The SECOM Years

I BECAME FOUNDING DEAN of the Southeastern College of Osteopathic Medicine (SECOM) in 1980; it was later to become Southeastern University of the Health Sciences. I stayed with that group until I retired in 1998 as Executive Vice Chancellor and Provost of the Health Professions Division of Nova Southeastern University (following our merger with Nova University). Even though some of the tales occurred in the 1980s, there were still signs of discrimination. Later tales show the progression toward acceptance and recognition, along with a couple of "interesting" stories that occurred during that period.

TALE 1

Hiring a Physiologist

ONE OF THE important tasks of a Founding Dean is to search for, hire and integrate the initial faculty. In some instances, we were successful—and lucky. One of our difficulties was in the hiring of our first physiologist.

We did an intensive search—first nationally and then locally. No luck. We had to fall back on Plan B: Hire a physiologist from a nearby university on a fee-for-service basis. Ultimately, we found such a person at the University of Miami School of Medicine and offered him a part-time fee-for-service teaching position.

However, he had to clear it with his superiors. Finally, it went to, I believe, the Dean's Council or the equivalent. The answer was a resounding "NO". In fact, the statement was made at that meeting that "SECOM is our competition." That professor could not be hired—even for the minor short time we needed. Fortunately, with increased activity and pressure, we were able to hire a young professor, Kenneth H. Woodside, PhD, who was hired as Chairman and turned out to be an excellent teacher and administrator. Our problem was solved. But a scar remained—the attitude of some administrators at U. of M.

Ultimately, and maybe it was stimulated by this episode, we enlisted the help of a fair-minded intermediary and he arranged a meeting of Mort Terry, me and Bernard Fogel, MD, dean of the medical school. From the start, Bernie was friendly, understanding, and cooperative. We parted on an amicable note—and from that point on, there was cooperation between the two institutions. Within a couple of years, we had become friendly enough that SECOM conferred an honorary degree on Dr. Fogel—something he accepted with joy.

Score another one for Osteopathic Medicine!

Tale 2

A "Different" Take on Discrimination

Many tales about discrimination are collected in this book. This one has a "different take" on the subject, one with a happy ending. This beautiful tale about discrimination—and the fear of it—occurred when I was dean of SECOM.

Cyril Blavo, DO, was a young black pediatrician with fine credentials, who applied for an opening in our College. My wife and I took him to dinner as part of his interview. He was friendly, cooperative and totally at ease. But when we left, I told my wife, "Something is strange here. I'm waiting for the other shoe to drop. He cannot be as good as he seems."

Fortunately, I knew his trainer well, so I called him. I told him of my concerns.

My friend, Stanley Grogg, DO, responded by saying, "Let me answer you with a story. Cyril was by far the best applicant we had for the residency. I also knew that in our hospital's clientele were a number of, well, "rednecks" and I just knew if they saw the color of Cyril's skin, they would probably never come back to our hospital. After much soul-searching, I decided that it was my responsibility to choose the best candidate—regardless of possible discrimination—so I appointed Cyril to the residency. And you know what, within three months, the "rednecks" would not let anyone except Cyril touch their children."

With that kind of recommendation, I was empowered to hire Cyril—and our experience was the same as Stan's. Satisfaction of his patients is universal. Patients love him and so do the parents. And he has been an academic treasure—from teaching Pediatrics to Pediatric practice to Director of our Master of Public Health program. He directs that division, with a full faculty, and among his many students is a large contingency of DO students taking a combined degree.

Cyril has been with us for more than 20 years. He is a fine example of what can happen when good people in a professional setting ignore discrimination—or the possibility of it.

Tale 3

Looking at Mergers

At one point in our growth, we thought that some sort of merger with another institution would be beneficial for us. Mort Terry had some brief talks with Nova University that went nowhere. Someone then suggested that we consider University of Miami. We had some mixed feelings. Probably it would be a good match but they were a giant against us. But we proceeded.

We moved in that direction, and were successful in arranging a combined meeting with some of UM's leaders and our leaders. It was to be a luncheon airing at our college for both parties. We had an auditorium but no great facilities for food service. And we did not have conference or banquet tables. So we set up a dozen or so 4-seat (bridge?) tables with no assigned seating.

Although there was some discussion and some informal remarks by a few leaders, one incident stands out in my mind—the only one I remember.

Sitting at my table was an Assistant Dean of the Medical School. There was some chatter, and then, softly, quietly, he said to me, "Why in the world would you want to merge with UM's medical school?"

I was nonplussed and the gentleman saw it in my face. He continued, "What you have built here and developed here in just a few short years, we could not do in tens of years." To me that made sense. While they were a giant operation that made progress slowly, we were a young organization, free of the complicating delays suffered by huge groups and we could do things in a hurry—no gradations of control, no financial interveners, none of those slowing-down steps characteristic of a bureaucratic institution. Of course, there was nothing negative about their educational system or their clinical operations but there was the usual giant administrative organization.

I immediately felt that this was not the right step. Dr. Terry, who was not sitting near me nor hearing this exchange, came to the same conclusion after all the discussion and side-bars.

So this possible merger went off the table. And I think it was the best thing. In fact, the President of UM vetoed the entire matter shortly thereafter, before we could announce our decision.

A couple of years later, I had the occasion to consult with the UM's then-Chairman of Neurology on a personal health matter. After the usual history and physical examination, he paused and said to me, "I know about the negotiations between you and UM. They were crazy not to want to merge with you, you guys have done such a marvelous job in so short a time."

Ah, more praise—and a feeling of accomplishment. More points for the osteopathic profession.

Tale 4

Student Stunts

Student admission interviews are a great source of stories—interesting, embarrassing, funny, the entire range. Here are two that remain stuck in my mind, even though I only participated in such interviews for the first few years of my deanship.

Applicant One was well past the middle of the interview when one interviewer—in spite of rules against such questions—asked him, "How do you expect to pay your tuition?"

Without missing a beat, the student replied, "My father has promised to pay all my tuition costs—I believe he has saved up the money. Plus that, my uncle, who is fairly wealthy, told me that if my father had any difficulty meeting the tuition, he would pay it."

Satisfied, the interview team went back to the regular routine. When it was finished, they thanked the student for coming in for the interview. The student responded by thanking the interview team and then, as he arose from his chair to leave, he turned back and asked, "Where is the Financial Aid Office?"

Applicant Two was slightly older than most applicants. The interview was going well until, in answering a question, he referenced "Dr. Neifield". Martin Neifield, DO, was a close personal friend of mine, plus he practiced in Philadelphia and did not come near South Florida—and the student lived and worked in Florida. Curious, and revealing nothing, I asked, "How do you know Dr. Neifield?"

The applicant was not flustered. His immediate answer was "I really don't know him personally, but his daughter told me I could use his name." Totally honest, and I think the committee appreciated that. And he was admitted. (By the way, Dr. Neifield's daughter had been a patient of mine for most of her formative years, so maybe I leaned in the student's direction.)

Yep, when you are interviewing applicants you should expect the unexpected, be prepared to get angry, or to feel compassion or to laugh. Both of these applicants created a laugh in the Admissions Committee.

Tale 5

Graduations

You plan and you plan and you plan. Then you schedule and schedule. Then you time it carefully. And if all goes well, you will have a successful graduation ceremony. Most of the time it works. But there are occasionally events that challenge your pattern. Those are the moments you most often remember.

Most of our graduations have gone well—but a few minor glitches occurred from time to time. And I do remember.

For our first graduation, my son and daughter-in-law surprised me with a visit from Philadelphia to attend, and, of course, they couldn't leave my new 3-month old grandchild home. I was certainly glad to see them. The processional went well. Everyone was seated and I, as the Dean, was the presiding officer. I stood up and walked to the podium. As I glanced down at the audience, I saw my family in the second row, and my daughter-in-law was breast-feeding Rachel. Talk about inhibiting moments. I'm sure it was only a few seconds delay but I remember it as a long inability to speak or open the ceremonies. Thank goodness, everything else went OK. Talk about speechless!

Our second graduation was held in a local auditorium. However, the dressing rooms were about a quarter-block from the auditorium. No problem. We planned it all out: how the processional lines would form, how to march from the dressing area, going outside to get to the auditorium and all such details. But we neglected just one thing. Five minutes before the march was scheduled, a tremendous downpour started (and continued for some time). So all of us—officials, guests, and the graduating class—got fully soaked and went into the auditorium drenched. Is it any solace to say that everything else went well? I can smile about it . . . now!

One scary situation occurred. Our routine for conferring degrees was to have someone call the alphabetical roll of the class and the graduates would walk to the stage to be hooded and receive their diplomas. Stan Cohen, EdD, one of our executive administrators, volunteered to call the list of 100 names. About half-way through, sudden silence; Stan fell to the floor—passed out. Of course there were a lot of physicians right on the stage and one or two of them jumped forward to take care of Stan while Marla Frohlinger, our Assistant Dean for Admissions and Student Affairs, immediately picked up Stan's list and continued almost without missing a beat. Stan was taken to the hospital and discharged a few hours later . . . in good health. So it all turned out OK.

Invocations, too, provide their share of worry—picking a clergyman, instructing him carefully about the five-minute limit and the absolute need for non-denominational service. One year we invited a local rabbi and went through all the instructions. He started his invocation beautifully . . . and went on . . . and on . . . and on . . . for 20 minutes. Needless to say, the entire stage party had mental, but silent, conniptions. But we survived.

One more invocation story. After we had almost exhausted the list of area clergymen, we decided to go to the graduating class for suggestions. We explained and asked them whether they had a preference or could suggest a name. One student raised her hand and said her father was a pastor and would be glad to do it. We grabbed at that opportunity—what a propitious coincidence. We went though the same instructions to the pastor. He delivered a beautiful message, and as he concluded he said, "This is Sunday, and if I were in my church right now, I would ask this in the name of the Father and the Son and the Holy Ghost." He sure delivered a non-denominational invocation but managed to satisfy us, and satisfy his own conscience, without offending anyone. What a brilliant move. And I told him so.

Graduations are a pleasant and satisfying affairs, for both staff and students. And, in spite of these few "memorable" occurrences, I enjoyed all 18 of them.

But, conscious or unconscious, there was a positive effect: hundreds of parents, relatives and friends—many being exposed for the first time—became impressed and osteopathic medicine picked up more recognition, perhaps additional understanding and many times, further support.

Tale 6

Starting a Pharmacy School

Some discrimination dies hard; this one was hidden but escaped, Early on, perhaps a year or two after the start of Southeastern College of Osteopathic Medicine, the Executive Director of Southeastern Medical Center (across the street from us) came to Dr. Morton Terry with a problem. He said that he had difficulty getting pharmacists, and thought part of the reason was that the only pharmacy school in Florida was located in the far north of the state.

That's all Mort Terry had to hear. He and I put our heads together and, with the splendid help of several local pharmacists, began to plan a pharmacy school. When word reached the University of Florida Pharmacy School (by the way, a fine institution), the Dean of the School addressed the faculty. He told them of our enterprise, and made the snide comment, "What are they going to teach—osteopathic pharmacy?"

It was not meant to be funny, but it was (to me at least). It also showed his attitude toward osteopathic medicine.

That little insult did not hold us back and within 15 months, we admitted our first pharmacy class. Pharmacy was our second school, followed by the College of Optometry, College of Allied Health, College of Medical Sciences, and eventually, the College of Dentistry.

The College of Pharmacy took off like a rocket and was a solid player in the Southeastern University of the Health Professions. Other schools were added, and ultimately, when we merged with Nova University, it all came under the rubric of the Health Professions Division of Nova Southeastern University.

We grew and developed. And never once did it interfere with or obstruct the U.F. Pharmacy School—and we found plenty of applicants who might not otherwise have achieved their dreams.

Yes, we taught osteopathic pharmacy—teach solid pharmacy subjects, collect the best faculty possible, and keep looking around for further opportunities to train young people in other health professions fields. And by spreading the word we were no longer just a small school for "quacks".

Besides gaining a pharmacy school, we gained positive exposure to every pharmacist in the state of Florida, their families and maybe their friends—and we continue to do so even today.

In spite of the vitriol against “osteopathic”, the establishment of a pharmacy school added to and enlarged the status of osteopathic medicine. It seems that every positive gain adds to the acceptance and reputation of our profession.

Tale 7

The Dental School

DENTISTRY AND OSTEOPATHIC Medicine?

At first bluish, it would create questions. But we were, after all, more than just a college of osteopathic medicine (with tentacles attached), we were the Division of Health Professions of the Nova Southeastern University. Rationale? All the health professions have a relationship with each other. Many of the subjects taught are duplicative, sometimes with different emphasis. In this sense, it was logical to look to dentistry as our next step.

We thought the idea sounded good. After all, there was only one dental school (and a good one) for the entire state of Florida and that was located in Gainseville, the far north of the state.

As we now had a wider scope for the Division, Mort Terry and I and our board felt that perhaps a little more intensive preparation was needed in considering a dental school. We put together a large Study Committee, and a representative one. We included Board members, faculty representatives, key administrators and several community dentists, all led by the Chairman, Seymour Oliet, DDS, a personal friend of mine who was Chairman of Endodontics at the University of Pennsylvania Dental School. They held a number of meetings and intensively discussed clinical, and practical, and philosophic aspects—and potential problems.

The Florida Dental Society and the American Dental Association raised interesting questions: Several dental schools had recently closed their doors (why would we succeed?), where are we going to get students (the application pool had diminished greatly) and where will we get patients if everyone who needs dental work can get it? Steven Zucker, DMD, head of our AHEC program, willingly undertook to study the problems presented—as a dentist and as a member of our administration. The committee considered all the questions and all of Steve's report and it unanimously recommended that we go ahead, so the College of Dental Medicine was established. And the NSU Board of Trustees, recognizing Dr. Oliet's dedication and ability, appointed him the founding Dean.

Suffice it to say that in each of those aspects, we have succeeded. Our application pool is one of the largest in the country, our clinics are loaded way beyond even the long waiting list and, perhaps, most important of all, since our founding, a number of new dental schools have been established in the United States or are in the process. Yes, an osteopathic college was the leader in the resurgence of dental education.

Our College of Osteopathic Medicine stands proudly alongside the College of Dental Medicine, as well as our four other health professions schools. And in the process, spreading the status of the osteopathic profession.

Tale 8

Council of Deans

Somewhere in the middle of my tenure as dean of SECOM, a meeting was convened in the state capitol of the deans of the four medical schools in the state of Florida—University of Florida, University of Miami, University of South Florida and SECOM. Several more meetings were held and it officially became the Council of Deans. We met two or three times a year to discuss mutual problems.

These meetings were friendly and without any signs of discrimination. At the start, there was no chairman and the meetings were sort of informal. After the first couple of meetings, the deans started to bring along a couple of Associate or Assistant Deans. Matthew Terry, DO, who was my Associate Dean, accompanied me to several of the meetings, and when I moved out of the deanship to become Vice President and Provost of the newly formed Southeastern University of the Health Sciences, Matt continued to represent us at the Council.

As I said, it was a very compatible group, even though I thought at times there were some hidden hostile feelings. My paranoia? Within a couple of years, Matt was elected Chairman of the Council, a sure sign of acceptance. And another first.

A few years later, Anthony Silvagni, DO, who followed Matt in our deanship, became active and eventually was also named Chairman of the Council. A far cry from the earlier years of rejection and non-acceptance. We had achieved a measure of state-wide recognition.

One meeting during my time with the Council still stands out in my mind, even though it occurred earlier. One of the other schools proposed a joint research project and it was discussed on the floor. I noted to the group that SECOM was a very young school and had no research programs or facilities. So, I proposed that the three schools proceed without us and we would lend any support we could.

The Dean of the UF school (who was "known" to be anti-osteopathic) was seated at the other end of the long conference table. He leaned forward and in very strong voice and manner said, "Arnold, we are <u>four</u> medical schools and anything we do, we will do together.

You must remain as part of this proposal." No discrimination here; it had gone or certainly diminished.

Everyone at the meeting agreed. That's where it stayed. "Anti-osteopathic" was gradually disappearing.

Tale 9

Our AHEC Program

One year when I was dean, I attended the annual meeting of the American Association of Colleges of Osteopathic Medicine (AACOM), and the featured speaker was Cherry Tsutsumida, head of the federal AHEC program (Area Health Education Centers). She described her interesting program, which concentrated on rural medicine and underserved populations, and provided additional training for medical students.

I listened aptly, as she listed the things that AHEC funded, taking it all in with glee. For, you see, we at SECOM were already doing a lot of what she outlined. Then and there, I decided we would go for an AHEC grant. We did not have grant writers and we had no prior experience with AHEC. I assigned the grant-writing to Stanley Cohen, EdD, who was our educational officer. Stan did a fine job and we were awarded a grant, the first one ever in Florida, and was one of the first ever given to any osteopathic institution (now there are a half-dozen.).

Unfortunately, the amount allotted, $180,000, was really small and we felt it was merely a token award. But we were pleased that we had broken the ice. We became the first osteopathic institution with an AHEC program; ultimately it developed into a major AHEC site—and further spread the reputation of Osteopathic Medicine, both among government officials and previously-uninformed citizens.

We started the work of integrating the monies we received with the programs we had already running. Shortly after that, the administrator we assigned as director of the AHEC program left our employ. We were fortunate that only a few weeks before, we had an application from an experienced AHEC administrator from up north—actually an Associate AHEC Director, so we immediately hired him. He was Steven Zucker, DMD, and he proved to be an outstanding head of our program.

Within weeks of getting our AHEC grant, we learned that the University of Miami was putting in an application for AHEC support for the following year. The general policy of AHEC at that time was to support only one program in each state. But we were quite willing to help our now-friendly neighbor. So Steve set about assisting UM where he could—and they did get a grant, unusual because of that unwritten rule. And they, too, developed a strong program. So now we had two AHECs in Florida. Over the years, both programs have continued to flourish and increase their grants every year.

Surprisingly, one day I received a phone call from Cherry Tsutsumida. She asked a favor:

Would I contact the University of Florida medical school and try to convince them to apply for an AHEC grant? Us? Li'l ole us? The osteopathic school? The tail wagging the dog? In a state already having two AHEC programs? Of course I did it, but without much result; actually, I was essentially told, "Don't call us; we'll call you." However, within a couple of years, and after seeing us develop so magnificently, they applied and were awarded a grant. Yes, three programs in one state! And SECOM was the lead group. Even the fourth Florida medical school, the University of South Florida, joined the ranks with an AHEC grant a couple of years later.

Beyond even that, there is no telling how much our program influenced other osteopathic institutions to create AHEC programs.

How far did this impact other people and communities? Some elementary statistics: well over 25,000 comunity-based AHEC student rotations (affecting many thousands of health professionals and patients); 5 million hours of service and learning in Florida's underserved communities; and over 200,000 school children, tobacco users and health professionals, all benefiting from AHEC programs. Outreach? With all that success, the name of the osteopathic profession spread widely. Similarly, the other osteopathic AHECs spread that influence throughout the country.

SECOM (now NSU-COM) is still a leader, and in 2012 we received $2.7 million in AHEC money and Dr. Zucker, who turned out to be one of the finest AHEC directors in the country, is justly proud of our total of about $75 million awarded to SECOM since we started with AHEC.

Such serendipity! And it started because we began our school with a constructive goal—and we had it operating.

But money is not the most important part of this. The resultant four AHEC programs have brought outstanding medical care to thousands who otherwise would be without it. And AHEC provided much-needed medical service to many rural and underserved areas. That's progress—and it started with an osteopathic college. And it actually helped bring the Florida medical schools together with collaborative efforts, a cooperation that enhanced the osteopathic profession's acceptance and recognition

So, the activity that we started spread, and with it, subtly but surely, the name and reputation of the osteopathic profession grew proportionately.

Tale 10

More Serendipity

MANY TIMES IN this book, I have pointed to serendipity as a factor in the advancement of Osteopathic Medicine. Or luck. Or good fortune. Or being in the right place at the right time.

That aphorism, freely translated in this example, means: being in the right place (or in a receptive condition) and then doing the right thing, practicing good medicine, providing patient-oriented care and consideration. When that good luck came our way, mostly we were ready for it—and ready to offer what the patients were looking for.

The growth of Southeastern College of Osteopathic Medicine as an institution is an example. From SECOM's founding in 1980, through the year 1996, we were in a constant state of growth (and it continues, though at a slower pace). Each time we added a class or increased the class size or developed a clinic or expanded a program, we extended SECOM's influence—and, without forethought, that of the osteopathic profession. Then, our expansion took a new direction: the founding of new health field schools.

Starting in the mid-eighties, we established five new health professions schools, all in record time, each established within 18 months of the concept being adopted. All of it covered a period of just over ten years. The added schools were:

College of Pharmacy. This was the first additional college, and it was widely known to be affiliated with an osteopathic college, even having interaction in their educational processes. Immediately, our "word" spread to the pharmacy profession all over the state—and in some instances, further than that. In addition, pharmacy faculty, whether they were otherwise knowledgeable or not about Osteopathic Medicine, became a part of the osteopathic world. And their families. And their community colleagues. And their friends. Similar phenomena happened when we established the other colleges.

College of Optometry. This was the first optometry school in Florida and one of only two in southern United States. Even though it was a separate and distinct college, it was known as a "sister" school to an osteopathic college and it opened new vistas for Osteopathic Medicine.

College of Allied Health. This school started with programs for Physician Assistant, Physical Therapy and Occupational Therapy, and it later added additional fields, including Nursing. Again, this exposed us to several new and entirely different audiences.

College of Medical Sciences. It provided the necessary basic science courses for all the other health schools, plus offering its own degrees in the basic science specialties.

College of Dental Medicine. This was the first new dental school in the U.S. in 25 years and only the second one in the state of Florida. These distinctions earned us—and Osteopathic Medicine—increased credibility.

That made five colleges in addition to the College of Osteopathic Medicine. Each move added a new sphere of influence and additional exposure for Osteopathic Medicine.

Then, SECOM, which had become Southeastern University of the Health Sciences, saw a greater opportunity. We merged with Nova University, a high-level university but without any health professions programs. We then became the Health Professions Division of the re-named Nova Southeastern University. Now we had additional exposure to a diverse university faculty and university students, plus the concomitant community of professions and people.

We never had a long-range plan for this expansion program. We never did this with an eye to increasing our exposure to greater populations, and certainly not (consciously) to increasing the advancement of Osteopathic Medicine. In fact, the topic or thought never came up but it was there, building step-by-step. We were there, developing complete and splendid patient care—and that was our goal. The rest followed. And Osteopathic Medicine advanced further. Without any forethought. Without any publicity. Without any hullabaloo.

And similar advancement of the osteopathic profession occurred with the establishment of every one of its new osteopathic colleges all over the country—another factor in the progress of Osteopathic Medicine. So many people, and institutions, to be grateful to.

Status of Osteopathic Medicine

2013

As the recognition and acceptance of the osteopathic profession grew—slowly at first, then phenomenally—so did the size of the profession, its students, its schools, its faculties. Or, perhaps the reverse: as the osteopathic profession underwent marked growth, so did its recognition and acceptance. Or, most likely, the two interacted together as both cause and effect.

The result was significant changes in the profession.

Medical Education. The standard timing remains intact today for both allopathic and osteopathic schools: almost universally, a four-year program divided equally into basic medical subjects and clinical experience. (A few schools in both branches have offered accelerated programs combining some undergraduate preparation and the full four-year medical curriculum.)

However, due to the marvelous advances in Medicine over the past 70 years and the accompanying growth of medical training. there is greater depth of teaching in both allopathic and osteopathic medical schools, and, in most cases, expansion of post-graduate training for specialties.

In terms of numbers, osteopathic education increased from 6 schools (1945) to a total today of 25 accredited schools with 30 locations (includes branch campuses). We are graduating almost 5,000 DOs every year, and our student population runs about 20,000. (It has been said that this year one out of every five medical school students will be a DO student, a phenomenal growth.) With this growth, our DO population in the United States has reached almost 80,000, of whom about 33% are females (with a student body including 46% females).

Faculties. In both schools of medicine, there has been important growths of faculty, both in size and in depth—just think about the important growth of sub-specialties across the professions. More and more today, our medical schools are using full-time faculty but often retaining some outside, part-time (visiting) faculty.

Post-Graduate. We now have about 25,000 DOs certified in specialties and sub-specialties, under the watchful eyes of 18 certifying boards. Every DO graduate who wants an osteopathic internship can get one. Those who want to go on may take an osteopathic specialty residency (there are presently 6,322 DOs in such programs)—and many DOs today are accepted into and serving in allopathic residencies.

Even the "old" General Practice—now called Family Practice—requires a residency and board certification. No more preceptorships!

Licensure. Today, every state in the country offers full, unrestricted licenses to practice medicine and surgery to all DO graduates.

Recognition and Acceptance. Today, DOs are almost universally accepted. We qualify for all positions in the Armed Forces, for all types of government positions, for Public Health Service jobs, and in most private situations. Today, DOs serve on the faculty of allopathic medical schools (some as department heads), are on the staffs of many allopathic hospitals (again, some as department chiefs) and in some of the most prestigious U.S. hospitals.

The best summary is the official current AMA definition of a physician "an individual who has received a 'Doctor of Medicine' or a 'Doctor of Osteopathic Medicine' degree or an equivalent degree following successful completion of a prescribed course of study from a school of medicine or osteopathic medicine."

We have come a long way in 70 years—in every aspect! And we must never forget that a major part of our success is the recognition accorded us by a continuously increasing public acceptance, backed up by the many dedicated and competent osteopathic physicians.

Epilogue

There you have it, my collection of osteopathic tales—stories, incidents, actions that occurred during the most expansive period in the history of the osteopathic profession (the 40s up to 2013). Some are purely interesting stories, others quite germane to our history and growth

In a manner, they represent happenings all over the United States, some draconian, some just serious, some light-hearted, some downright funny. I make no claim for exclusivity—I know that similar stories and events were taking places across the country during the same period. Thousands of my colleagues experienced them but may not have recorded them. But each victory opened another advance—or two—or three.

Perhaps it is too simple to say that the osteopathic profession as a group went from the beginning of the century being rejected, unrecognized, and unaccepted to the end of the century with most of those difficulties gone.

I believe that the fantastic progress and growth of the osteopathic profession were brought about by a few major things:

Thousand of individual DOs interacting with the allopathic medical system, practicing and demonstrating excellent medical care (in spite of oppression). They converted medical enemies to friends and inch-by-inch improved the acceptance of osteopathic medicine. Some did it by seeking formal graduate training, some by becoming affiliates (outside the walls) of allopathic institutions. None of us said, "I will now do such-and-such to improve acceptance of my profession." We—thousands like me—did it by doing the right things every day and in every way

The development of osteopathic hospitals, with its concomitant (and needed) expansion of specialists—and enlarging the number of osteopathic specialists. Many of these hospitals started on a shoe-string just to give DOs a local hospital in which to take care of their patients. As specialists' numbers increased, their respective osteopathic specialty organizations grew, becoming stronger and stronger—and spreading the word.

The work of many osteopathic organizations, active in seeking recognition when there were legal or quasi-legal blockages—or where there were unfulfilled opportunities. One of the major ones was the opening of medical commissions in the armed services to DOs. Subsequent to this, other government medical positions—federal and state and local—became available to osteopathic physicians. At the same time these osteopathic organizations were providing positive publicity about the osteopathic profession by their professional demeanor, practice and activity. Throughout all this, the American Osteopathic Association led the fight, bringing about much of the progress, especially with governmental groups, while continuously acquainting the public with Osteopathic Medicine. These osteopathic organizations grew as the profession grew.

The phenomenal growth of the osteopathic profession. Our osteopathic population grew from 9,500 DOs in the United States in 1940 to almost 80,000 today, adding numerical strength to the advancement struggle. (Consider even just the single concept of more than eight times the number of DOs contacting the public and other professions daily.) In this, we must express gratitude to the original few osteopathic colleges who increased their enrollments and to the new schools, who together are rapidly producing more and more DOs while maintaining high academic standards. In fact, total enrollment in our colleges went from several hundred students in 1940 to over 20,000 today, with 6000 post-doctoral residency slots.

Thousands of DOs from Andrew Taylor Still to today's DOs who advanced our profession by conscientious practice and by providing high-quality care in treating and curing patients every day of the week. Most of them, while staying true to the A.T. Still beginnings, followed and accepted applicable modern scientific medicine, actually drifting slowly into the mainstream of medicine and bringing their patients the best possible care.

The cooperation of MDs. We cannot overlook those important early MDs who cooperated in this progress by their work with osteopathic physicians—no, not primarily to advance the osteopathic profession, but because it would help patients and serve Medicine. And also we must remember the thousands of additional MDs who have since come aboard in this giant venture.

No one person—or two or three—can be credited with the rise of Osteopathic Medicine. Andrew Taylor Still, alone, founded the profession, but it took thousands of DOs in the intervening years, to bring us to today's status.

To all of them, we all owe a great debt of gratitude. We have eliminated most of the discrimination, and we can now move on to positive goals.

For my part, I thank them profusely and I am grateful and indebted for the opportunity of living through and being active in the progress of the last 70 years. With all my heart, I thank all those who were a part of it.

Thus endeth my tales, but what a rosy future!

www.ingramcontent.com/pod-product-compliance
Lightning Source LLC
Chambersburg PA
CBHW032012170526
45157CB00002B/657
* 9 7 8 1 4 8 1 7 3 2 2 4 6 *